DASH DIET COOKBOOK

2022

EASY AND FLAVORFUL RECIPES TO SPEED WEIGHT LOSS AND PREVENT DIABETES

HANNA PORTER

Table of Contents

Peanut Butter Oats 12

Scones with Nuts and Fruits 13

Banana Cookies 14

Apple Oats 15

Blueberry Muffins 16

Coconut Crepes 18

Blueberry Pancakes 19

Pumpkin Parfait 20

Sweet Potato Waffles 21

French Toast 22

Cocoa Oats 23

Mango Oatmeal 24

Cherries and Pears Oatmeal 25

Pecan and Orange Bowls 26

Baked Peaches and Cream 27

Apples and Yogurt Bowls 28

Mango and Pomegranate Oatmeal 29

Chia Seeds and Pomegranate Bowls 30

Egg and Carrots Hash 31

Bell Peppers Omelet 32

Parsley Frittata 33

Baked Eggs and Artichokes 34

Beans and Eggs Casserole 35

Turmeric Cheesy Scramble 36

Hash Browns and Veggies	37
Chives Bacon Risotto	39
Cinnamon Pistachio Quinoa	40
Cherries Yogurt Mix	41
Plums and Coconut Mix	42
Apples Yogurt	43
Strawberry and Oats Bowls	44
Maple Peach Mix	45
Cinnamon Rice and Dates	46
Figs, Pear and Pomegranate Yogurt	47
Nutmeg Strawberry Porridge	48
Creamy Rice and Berries	49
Vanilla Coconut Rice	50
Coconut Rice and Cherries	51
Ginger Rice Mix	52
Chili Sausage Casserole	53
Mushroom Rice Bowls	54
Tomato and Spinach Eggs	55
Sesame Omelet	56
Zucchini Oatmeal	57
Almonds and Coconut Bowl	58
Warm Chickpeas Salad	59
Cocoa Millet Pudding	60
Chia Pudding	61
Tapioca Pudding	62
Cheddar Hash	63
Snow Peas Salad	64

- Quinoa and Chickpeas Mix 65
- Olives and Peppers Salad 66
- Green Beans and Eggs Mix 67
- Carrot and Eggs Salad.. 68
- Creamy Berries 69
- Apples and Raisins Bowls 70
- Ginger Buckwheat Porridge... 71
- Cauliflower and Peppers Salad 72
- Chicken and Hash Browns 73

Dash Diet Lunch Recipes 74

- Black Beans Burritos 75
- Chicken and Mango Mix.. 76
- Chickpeas Cakes.. 77
- Salsa and Cauliflower Bowls 78
- Salmon and Spinach Salad 79
- Chicken and Kale Mix 80
- Salmon and Arugula Salad.. 81
- Shrimp and Veggies Salad 82
- Turkey and Peppers Wraps 83
- Green Beans Soup... 84
- Avocado, Spinach and Olives Salad.. 85
- Beef and Zucchini Pan 86
- Thyme Beef and Potatoes Mix.. 87
- Pork and Carrots Soup 88
- Shrimp and Strawberry Salad 89
- Shrimp and Green Beans Salad... 90
- Fish Tacos 91

Zucchini Cakes	92
Chickpeas and Tomatoes Stew	93
Chicken, Tomato and Spinach Salad	94
Asparagus and Peppers Bowls	95
Hot Beef Stew	96
Pork Chops with Mushrooms	97
Coriander Shrimp Salad	98
Eggplant Stew	99
Beef and Peas Mix	100
Turkey Stew	101
Beef Salad	102
Squash Stew	104
Cabbage and Beef Mix	105
Pork and Green Beans Stew	106
Zucchini Cream Soup	107
Shrimp and Grapes Salad	108
Turmeric Carrot Cream	109
Beef and Black Beans Soup	110
Salmon and Shrimp Bowls	111
Chicken and Garlic Sauce	112
Turmeric Chicken and Eggplant Stew	113
Chicken and Endives Mix	114
Turkey Soup	115
Shrimp and Pineapple mix	116
Salmon and Green Olives	117
Salmon and Fennel	118
Cod and Asparagus	119

Spiced Shrimp	120
Sea Bass and Tomatoes	121
Shrimp and Beans	122
Shrimp and Horseradish Mix	123
Shrimp and Tarragon Salad	124
Parmesan Cod Mix	125
Tilapia and Red Onion Mix	126
Trout Salad	127
Balsamic Trout	128
Parsley Salmon	129
Trout and Veggie Salad	130
Saffron Salmon	131
Shrimp and Watermelon Salad	132
Oregano Shrimp and Quinoa Salad	133
Crab Salad	134
Balsamic Scallops	135
Creamy Flounder Mix	136
Spicy Salmon and Mango Mix	137
Dill Shrimp Mix	138
Salmon Pate	139
Shrimp with Artichokes	140
Shrimp with Lemon Sauce	141
Tuna and Orange Mix	142
Salmon Curry	143
Salmon and Carrots Mix	144
Shrimp and Pine Nuts Mix	145
Chili Cod and Green Beans	146

- Garlic Scallops ... 147
- Creamy Sea Bass Mix ... 148
- Sea Bass and Mushrooms Mix ... 149
- Salmon Chowder ... 150
- Nutmeg Shrimp ... 151
- Shrimp and Berries Mix ... 152
- Baked Lemony Trout ... 153
- Chives Scallops ... 154
- Tuna Meatballs ... 155
- Salmon Pan ... 156
- Mustard Cod Mix ... 157
- Shrimp and Asparagus Mix ... 158
- Cod and Peas ... 159
- Shrimp and Mussels Bowls ... 160

Dash Diet Dessert Recipes ... 161
- Mint Cream ... 162
- Raspberries Pudding ... 163
- Almond Bars ... 164
- Baked Peaches Mix ... 165
- Walnuts Cake ... 166
- Apple Cake ... 167
- Cinnamon Cream ... 168
- Creamy Strawberries Mix ... 169
- Vanilla Pecan Brownies ... 170
- Strawberries Cake ... 171
- Cocoa Pudding ... 173
- Nutmeg Vanilla Cream ... 174

Avocado Cream	175
Raspberries Cream	176
Watermelon Salad	177
Coconut Pears Mix	178
Apples Compote	179
Apricots Stew	180
Lemon Cantaloupe Mix	181
Creamy Rhubarb Cream	182
Pineapple Bowls	183
Blueberry Stew	184
Lime Pudding	185
Peach Cream	186
Cinnamon Plums Mix	187
Chia and Vanilla Apples	188
Rice and Pears Pudding	189
Rhubarb Stew	190
Rhubarb Cream	191
Blueberries Salad	192
Dates and Banana Cream	193
Plum Muffins	194
Plums and Raisins Bowls	195
Sunflower Seed Bars	196
Blackberries and Cashews Bowls	197
Orange and Mandarins Bowls	198
Pumpkin Cream	199
Figs and Rhubarb Mix	200
Spiced Banana	201

Cocoa Smoothie 202

Banana Bars 203

Green Tea and Dates Bars 204

Walnut Cream 205

Lemon Cake 206

Raisins Bars 207

Nectarines Squares 208

Grapes Stew 209

Mandarin and Plums Cream 210

Cherry and Strawberries Cream... 211

Cardamom Walnuts and Rice Pudding 212

Pears Bread 213

Rice and Cherries Pudding 214

Watermelon Stew 215

Ginger Pudding 216

Cashew Cream 217

Hemp Cookies 218

Almonds and Pomegranate Bowls 219

Peanut Butter Oats

Preparation time: 6 hours and 10 minutes

Cooking time: 0 minutes
Servings: 1

Ingredients:
- 1 tablespoon chia seeds
- ½ cup almond milk
- 2 tablespoons natural peanut butter
- 1 tablespoon stevia
- ½ cup gluten-free oats
- 2 tablespoons raspberries

Directions:
1. In a mason jar, combine the oats with the chia seeds and the other ingredients except the raspberries, stir a bit, cover and keep in the fridge for 6 hours.
2. Top with the raspberries and serve for breakfast.

Nutrition: calories 454, fat 23.9, fiber 12, carbs 50.9, protein 14.6

Scones with Nuts and Fruits

Preparation time: 10 minutes
Cooking time: 12 minutes
Servings: 8

Ingredients:
- 2 cups almond flour
- ½ teaspoon baking soda
- ¼ cup cranberries, dried
- ¼ cup sunflower seeds
- ¼ cup apricots, chopped
- ¼ cup walnuts, chopped
- ¼ cup sesame seeds
- 2 tablespoons stevia
- 1 egg, whisked

Directions:
1. In a bowl, combine the flour with the baking soda, cranberries and the other ingredients and stir well.
2. Shape a square dough, roll onto a floured working surface and cut into 16 squares.
3. Arrange the squares on a baking sheet lined with parchment paper and bake the scones at 350 degrees F for 12 minutes.
4. Serve the scones for breakfast.

Nutrition: calories 238, fat 19.2, fiber 4.1, carbs 8.6, protein 8.8

Banana Cookies

Preparation time: 10 minutes
Cooking time: 15 minutes
Servings: 12

Ingredients:
- 1 cup almond butter
- ¼ cup stevia
- 1 teaspoon vanilla extract
- 2 bananas, peeled and mashed
- 2 cups gluten-free oats
- 1 teaspoon cinnamon powder
- 1 cup almonds, chopped
- ½ cup raisins

Directions:
1. In a bowl, combine the butter with the stevia and the other ingredients and stir well using a hand mixer.
2. Scoop medium moulds of this mix on a baking sheet lined with parchment paper and flatten them a bit.
3. Cook them at 325 degrees F for 15 minutes and serve for breakfast.

Nutrition: calories 280, fat 16, fiber 4, carbs 29, protein 8

Apple Oats

Preparation time: 10 minutes
Cooking time: 7 hours
Servings: 4

Ingredients:
- 2 apples, cored, peeled and cubed
- 1 cup gluten-free oats
- 1 and ½ cups water
- 1 and ½ cups almond milk
- 2 tablespoons swerve
- 2 tablespoons almond butter
- ½ teaspoon cinnamon powder
- 1 tablespoon flax seed, ground
- Cooking spray

Directions:
1. Grease a slow cooker with the cooking spray and combine the oats with the water and the other ingredients inside.
2. Toss a bit and cook on Low for 7 hours.
3. Divide into bowls and serve for breakfast.

Nutrition: calories 149, fat 3.6, fiber 3.9, carbs 27.3, protein 4.9

Blueberry Muffins

Preparation time: 10 minutes
Cooking time: 25 minutes
Servings: 12

Ingredients:
- 2 bananas, peeled and mashed
- 1 cup almond milk
- 1 teaspoon vanilla extract
- ¼ cup pure maple syrup
- 1 teaspoon apple cider vinegar
- ¼ cup coconut oil, melted
- 2 cups almond flour
- 4 tablespoons coconut sugar
- 2 teaspoons cinnamon powder
- 2 teaspoons baking powder
- 2 cups blueberries
- ½ teaspoon baking soda
- ½ cup walnuts, chopped

Directions:
1. In a bowl, combine the bananas with the almond milk, vanilla and the other ingredients and whisk well.
2. Divide the mix into 12 muffin tins and bake at 350 degrees F for 25 minutes.
3. Serve the muffins for breakfast.

Nutrition: calories 180,, fat 5, fiber 2, carbs 31, protein 4

Coconut Crepes

Preparation time: 10 minutes
Cooking time: 6 minutes
Servings: 12

Ingredients:
- 1 cup almond flour
- 1 tablespoon flaxseed, ground
- 2 cups coconut milk
- 2 tablespoons coconut oil, melted
- 1 teaspoon cinnamon powder
- 2 teaspoons stevia

Directions:
1. In a bowl, combine the flour with the flaxseed, milk, half of the oil, cinnamon and stevia and whisk well.
2. Heat up a pan with the rest of the oil over medium heat, add ¼ cup of the crepes batter, spread into the pan, cook for 2-3 minutes on each side and transfer to a plate.
3. Repeat with the rest of the crepes batter and serve them for breakfast.

Nutrition: calories 71, fat 3, fiber 1, carbs 8, protein 1

Blueberry Pancakes

Preparation time: 10 minutes
Cooking time: 7 minutes
Servings: 12

Ingredients:
- 2 eggs, whisked
- 4 tablespoons almond milk
- 1 cup full-fat yogurt
- 3 tablespoons coconut butter, melted
- ½ teaspoon vanilla extract
- 1 and ½ cups almond flour
- 2 tablespoons stevia
- 1 cup blueberries
- 1 tablespoon avocado oil

Directions:
1. In a bowl, combine the eggs with the almond milk and the other ingredients except the oil and whisk well.
2. Heat up a pan with the oil over medium heat, add ¼ cup of the batter, spread into the pan, cook for 4 minutes, flip, cook for 3 minutes more and transfer to a plate.
3. Repeat with the rest of the batter and serve the pancakes for breakfast.

Nutrition: calories 64, fat 4.4, fiber 1.1, carbs 4.7, protein 1.8

Pumpkin Parfait

Preparation time: 10 minutes
Cooking time: 0 minutes
Servings: 4

Ingredients:
- ¼ cup cashews
- ½ cup water
- 2 teaspoons pumpkin pie spice
- 2 cups pumpkin puree
- 2 tablespoons maple syrup
- 1 pear, cored, peeled and chopped
- 2 cups coconut yogurt

Directions:
1. In a blender, combine the cashews with the water and the other ingredients except the yogurt and pulse well.
2. Divide the yogurt into bowls, also divide the pumpkin cream on top and serve.

Nutrition: calories 200, fat 6.4, fiber 5.1, carbs 32.9, protein 5.5

Sweet Potato Waffles

Preparation time: 10 minutes
Cooking time: 10 minutes
Servings: 6

Ingredients:
- ½ cup sweet potato, cooked, peeled and grated
- 1 cup almond milk
- 1 cup gluten-free oats
- 2 eggs, whisked
- 1 tablespoon honey
- ¼ teaspoon baking powder
- 1 tablespoon olive oil
- Cooking spray

Directions:
1. In a bowl, combine the sweet potato with the almond milk and the rest of the ingredients except the cooking spray and whisk well.
2. Grease the waffle iron with the cooking spray and pour 1/3 of the batter in each mould.
3. Cook the waffles for 3-4 minutes and serve them for breakfast.

Nutrition: calories 352, fat 22.4, fiber 6.7, carbs 33.4, protein 8.4

French Toast

Preparation time: 10 minutes
Cooking time: 5 minutes
Servings: 2

Ingredients:

- 4 whole wheat bread slices
- 2 tablespoons coconut sugar
- ½ cup coconut milk
- 2 eggs, whisked
- 1 teaspoon vanilla extract
- Cooking spray

Directions:

1. In a bowl, combine the sugar with the milk, eggs and the vanilla and whisk well.
2. Dip each bread slice in this mix.
3. Heat up a pan greased with cooking spray over medium heat, add the French toast, cook for 2-3 minutes on each side, divide between plates and serve for breakfast.

Nutrition: calories 508, fat 30.8, fiber 7.1, carbs 55.1, protein 16.2

Cocoa Oats

Preparation time: 10 minutes
Cooking time: 20 minutes
Servings: 4

Ingredients:
- 2 cups almond milk
- 1 cup old-fashioned oats
- 2 tablespoons coconut sugar
- 1 teaspoon cocoa powder
- 2 teaspoons vanilla extract

Directions:
1. Heat up a pot with the milk over medium heat, add the oats and the other ingredients, bring to a simmer and cook for 20 minutes.
2. Divide the oats into bowls and serve warm for breakfast.

Nutrition: calories 406, fat 30, fiber 4.8, carbs 30.2, protein 6

Mango Oatmeal

Preparation time: 10 minutes
Cooking time: 20 minutes
Servings: 4

Ingredients:
- 2 cups coconut milk
- 1 cup old-fashioned oats
- 1 cup mango, peeled and cubed
- 3 tablespoons almond butter
- 2 tablespoons coconut sugar
- ½ teaspoon vanilla extract

Directions:
1. Put the milk in a pot, heat it up over medium heat, add the oats and the other ingredients, stir, bring to a simmer and cook for 20 minutes.
2. Stir the oatmeal, divide it into bowls and serve.

Nutrition: calories 531, fat 41.8, fiber 7.5, carbs 42.7, protein 9.3

Cherries and Pears Oatmeal

Preparation time: 10 minutes
Cooking time: 10 minutes
Servings: 6

Ingredients:
- 2 cups old-fashioned oats
- 3 cups almond milk
- 2 and ½ tablespoons cocoa powder
- 1 teaspoon vanilla extract
- 10 ounces cherries, pitted
- 2 pears, cored, peeled and cubed

Directions:
1. In your pressure cooker, combine the oats with the milk and the other ingredients, toss, cover and cook on High for 10 minutes.
2. Release the pressure naturally for 10 minutes, stir the oatmeal one more time, divide it into bowls and serve.

Nutrition: calories 477, fat 30.7, fiber 8.3, carbs 49.6, protein 7

Pecan and Orange Bowls

Preparation time: 10 minutes
Cooking time: 20 minutes
Servings: 4

Ingredients:
- 1 cup steel cut oats
- 2 cups orange juice
- 2 tablespoons coconut butter, melted
- 2 tablespoons stevia
- 3 tablespoons pecans, chopped
- ¼ teaspoon vanilla extract

Directions:
1. Heat up a pot with the orange juice over medium heat, add the oats, the butter and the other ingredients, whisk, simmer for 20 minutes, divide into bowls and serve for breakfast.

Nutrition: calories 288, fat 39.1, fiber 3.4, carbs 48.3, protein 4.7

Baked Peaches and Cream

Preparation time: 10 minutes
Cooking time: 20 minutes
Servings: 4

Ingredients:
- 2 cups coconut cream
- 1 teaspoon cinnamon powder
- 1/3 cup palm sugar
- 4 peaches, stones removed and cut into wedges
- Cooking spray

Directions:
1. Grease a baking pan with the cooking spray and combine the peaches with the other ingredients inside.
2. Bake this at 360 degrees F for 20 minutes, divide into bowls and serve for breakfast.

Nutrition: calories 338, fat 29.2, fiber 4.9, carbs 21, protein 4.2

Apples and Yogurt Bowls

Preparation time: 10 minutes
Cooking time: 15 minutes
Servings: 4

Ingredients:
- 1 cup steel cut oats
- 1 and ½ cups almond milk
- 1 cup non-fat yogurt
- ¼ cup maple syrup
- 2 apples, cored, peeled and chopped
- ½ teaspoon cinnamon powder

Directions:
1. In a pot, combine the oats with the m ilk and the other ingredients except the yogurt, toss, bring to a simmer and cook over medium-high heat for 15 minutes.
2. Divide the yogurt into bowls, divide the apples and oats mix on top and serve for breakfast.

Nutrition: calories 490, fat 30.2, fiber 7.4, carbs 53.9, protein 7

Mango and Pomegranate Oatmeal

Preparation time: 10 minutes
Cooking time: 20 minutes
Servings: 4

Ingredients:
- 3 cups almond milk
- 1 cup steel cut oats
- 1 tablespoon cinnamon powder
- 1 mango, peeled, and cubed
- ½ teaspoon vanilla extract
- 3 tablespoons pomegranate seeds

Directions:
1. Put the milk in a pot and heat it up over medium heat.
2. Add the oats, cinnamon and the other ingredients, toss, simmer for 20 minutes, divide into bowls and serve for breakfast.

Nutrition: calories 568, fat 44.6, fiber 7.5, carbs 42.5, protein 7.8

Chia Seeds and Pomegranate Bowls

Preparation time: 10 minutes
Cooking time: 20 minutes
Servings: 4

Ingredients:
- ½ cup steel cut oats
- 2 cups almond milk
- ¼ cup pomegranate seeds
- 4 tablespoons chia seeds
- 1 teaspoon vanilla extract

Directions:
1. Put the milk in a pot, bring to a simmer over medium heat, add the oats and the other ingredients, bring to a simmer and cook for 20 minutes.
2. Divide the mix into bowls and serve for breakfast.

Nutrition: calories 462, fat 38, fiber 13.5, carbs 27.1, protein 8.8

Egg and Carrots Hash

Preparation time: 10 minutes
Cooking time: 20 minutes
Servings: 4

Ingredients:
- 2 carrots, peeled and cubed
- 1 tablespoon olive oil
- 1 yellow onion, chopped
- 1 cup low-fat cheddar cheese, shredded
- 8 eggs, whisked
- 1 cup coconut milk
- A pinch of salt and black pepper

Directions:
1. Heat up a pan with the oil over medium heat, add the onion and the carrots, toss and brown for 5 minutes.
2. Add the eggs and the other ingredients, toss, cook for 15 minutes stirring often, divide between plates and serve.

Nutrition: calories 431, fat 35.9, fiber 2.7, carbs 10, protein 20

Bell Peppers Omelet

Preparation time: 10 minutes
Cooking time: 15 minutes
Servings: 4

Ingredients:
- 4 eggs, whisked
- A pinch of black pepper
- ¼ cup low-sodium bacon, chopped
- 1 tablespoons olive oil
- 1 cup red bell peppers, chopped
- 4 spring onions, chopped
- ¾ cup low-fat cheese, shredded

Directions:
1. Heat up a pan with the oil over medium heat, add the spring onions and the bell peppers, toss and cook for 5 minutes.
2. Add the eggs and the other ingredients, toss, spread into the pan, cook for 5 minutes, flip, cook for another 5 minutes, divide between plates and serve.

Nutrition: calories 288, fat 18, fiber 0.8, carbs 4, protein 13.4

Parsley Frittata

Preparation time: 10 minutes
Cooking time: 20 minutes
Servings: 4

Ingredients:
- A pinch of black pepper
- 4 eggs, whisked
- 2 tablespoons parsley, chopped
- 1 tablespoon low-fat cheese, shredded
- 1 red onion, chopped
- 1 tablespoon olive oil

Directions:
1. Heat up a pan with the oil over medium heat, add the onion and the black pepper, stir and sauté for 5 minutes.
2. Add the eggs mixed with the other ingredients, spread into the pan, introduce in the oven and cook at 360 degrees F for 15 minutes.
3. Divide the frittata between plates and serve.

Nutrition: calories 112, fat 8.5, fiber 0.7, carb 3.1, protein 6.3

Baked Eggs and Artichokes

Preparation time: 5 minutes
Cooking time: 20 minutes
Servings: 4

Ingredients:
- 4 eggs
- 4 slices low-fat cheddar, shredded
- 1 yellow onion, chopped
- 1 tablespoon avocado oil
- 1 tablespoon cilantro, chopped
- 1 cup canned no-salt-added artichokes, drained and chopped

Directions:
1. Grease 4 ramekins with the oil, divide the onion in each, crack an egg in each ramekin, add the artichokes and top with cilantro and cheddar cheese.
2. Introduce the ramekins in the oven and bake at 380 degrees F for 20 minutes.
3. Serve the baked eggs for breakfast.

Nutrition: calories 178, fat 10.9, fiber 2.9, carbs 8.4, protein 14.2

Beans and Eggs Casserole

Preparation time: 10 minutes
Cooking time: 30 minutes
Servings: 8

Ingredients:
- 8 eggs, whisked
- 2 red onions, chopped
- 1 red bell pepper, chopped
- 4 ounces canned black beans, no-salt-added, drained and rinsed
- ½ cup green onions, chopped
- 1 cup low-fat mozzarella cheese, shredded
- Cooking spray

Directions:
1. Grease a baking pan with the cooking spray and spread the black beans, onions, green onions and bell pepper into the pan.
2. Add the eggs mixed with the cheese, introduce in the oven and bake at 380 degrees F for 30 minutes.
3. Divide the mix between plates and serve for breakfast.

Nutrition: calories 140, fat 4.7, fiber 3.4, carbs 13.6, protein 11.2

Turmeric Cheesy Scramble

Preparation time: 10 minutes
Cooking time: 15 minutes
Servings: 4

Ingredients:
- 3 tablespoons low-fat mozzarella, shredded
- A pinch of black pepper
- 4 eggs, whisked
- 1 red bell pepper, chopped
- 1 teaspoon turmeric powder
- 1 tablespoon olive oil
- 2 shallots, chopped

Directions:
1. Heat up a pan with the oil over medium heat, add the shallots and the bell pepper, stir and sauté for 5 minutes.
2. Add the eggs mixed with the rest of the ingredients, stir, cook for 10 minutes, divide everything between plates and serve.

Nutrition: calories 138, fat 8, fiber 1.3, carbs 4.6, protein 12

Hash Browns and Veggies

Preparation time: 10 minutes
Cooking time: 20 minutes
Servings: 4

Ingredients:
- 1 tablespoon olive oil
- 4 eggs, whisked
- 1 cup hash browns
- ½ cup fat-free cheddar cheese, shredded
- 1 small yellow onion, chopped
- A pinch of black pepper
- ½ green bell pepper, chopped
- ½ red bell pepper, chopped
- 1 carrot, chopped
- 1 tablespoon cilantro, chopped

Directions:
1. Heat up a pan with the oil over medium-high heat, add the onion and the hash browns and cook for 5 minutes.
2. Add the bell peppers and the carrots, toss and cook for 5 minutes more.
3. Add the eggs, black pepper and the cheese, stir and cook for another 10 minutes.
4. Add the cilantro, stir, cook for a couple more seconds, divide everything between plates and serve for breakfast.

Nutrition: calories 277, fat 17.5, fiber 2.7, carbs 19.9, protein 11

Chives Bacon Risotto

Preparation time: 10 minutes
Cooking time: 25 minutes
Servings: 4

Ingredients:
- 3 slices bacon, low-sodium, chopped
- 1 tablespoon avocado oil
- 1 cup white rice
- 1 red onion, chopped
- 2 cups low-sodium chicken stock
- 2 tablespoons low-fat parmesan, grated
- 1 tablespoon chives, chopped
- A pinch of black pepper

Directions:
1. Heat up a pan with the oil over medium-high heat, add the onion and the bacon, stir and cook for 5 minutes.
2. Add the rice and the other ingredients, toss, bring to a simmer and cook over medium heat for 20 minutes.
3. Stir the mix, divide into bowls and serve for breakfast.

Nutrition: calories 271, fat 7.2, fiber 1.4, carbs 40, protein 9.9

Cinnamon Pistachio Quinoa

Preparation time: 5 minutes
Cooking time: 10 minutes
Servings: 4

Ingredients:
- 1 and ½ cups water
- 1 teaspoon cinnamon powder
- 1 and ½ cups quinoa
- 1 cup almond milk
- 1 tablespoon coconut sugar
- ¼ cup pistachios, chopped

Directions:
1. Put the water and the almond milk in a pot, bring to a boil over medium heat, add the quinoa and the other ingredients, whisk, cook for 10 minutes, divide in to bowls, cool down and serve for breakfast.

Nutrition: calories 222, fat 16.7, fiber 2.5, carbs 16.3, protein 3.9

Cherries Yogurt Mix

Preparation time: 10 minutes
Cooking time: 0 minutes
Servings: 4

Ingredients:
- 4 cups non-fat yogurt
- 1 cup cherries, pitted and halved
- 4 tablespoons coconut sugar
- ½ teaspoon vanilla extract

Directions:
1. In a bowl, combine the yogurt with the cherries, sugar and vanilla, toss and keep in the fridge for 10 minutes.
2. Divide into bowls and serve f breakfast.

Nutrition: calories 145, fat 0, fiber 0.1, carbs 29, protein 2.3

Plums and Coconut Mix

Preparation time: 10 minutes
Cooking time: 15 minutes
Servings: 4

Ingredients:
- 4 plums, pitted and halved
- 3 tablespoons coconut oil, melted
- ½ teaspoon cinnamon powder
- 1 cup coconut cream
- ¼ cup unsweetened coconut, shredded
- 2 tablespoons sunflower seeds, toasted

Directions:
1. In a baking dish, combine the plums with the oil, cinnamon and the other ingredients, introduce in the oven and bake at 380 degrees F for 15 minutes.
2. Divide everything into bowls and serve.

Nutrition: calories 282, fat 27.1, fiber 2.8, carbs 12.4, protein 2.3

Apples Yogurt

Preparation time: 10 minutes
Cooking time: 0 minutes
Servings: 4

Ingredients:
- 6 apples, cored and pureed
- 1 cup natural apple juice
- 2 tablespoons coconut sugar
- 2 cups non-fat yogurt
- 1 teaspoon cinnamon powder

Directions:
1. In a bowl, combine the apples with the apple juice and the other ingredients, stir, divide into bowls and keep in the fridge for 10 minutes before serving.

Nutrition: calories 289, fat 0.6, fiber 8.7, carbs 68.5, protein 3.9

Strawberry and Oats Bowls

Preparation time: 10 minutes
Cooking time: 20 minutes
Servings: 4

Ingredients:
- 1 and ½ cups gluten-free oats
- 2 and ¼ cups almond milk
- ½ teaspoon vanilla extract
- 2 cups strawberries, sliced
- 2 tablespoons coconut sugar

Directions:
1. Put the milk in a pot, bring to a simmer over medium heat, add the oats and the other ingredients, stir, cook for 20 minutes, divide into bowls and serve for breakfast.

Nutrition: calories 216, fat 1.5, fiber 3.4, carbs 39.5, protein 10.4

Maple Peach Mix

Preparation time: 10 minutes
Cooking time: 15 minutes
Servings: 4

Ingredients:
- 4 peaches, cored and cut into wedges
- ¼ cup maple syrup
- ¼ teaspoon almond extract
- ½ cup almond milk

Directions:
1. Put the almond milk in a pot, bring to a simmer over medium heat, add the peaches and the other ingredients, toss, cook for 15 minutes, divide into bowls and serve for breakfast.

Nutrition: calories 180, fat 7.6, fiber 3, carbs 28.9, protein 2.1

Cinnamon Rice and Dates

Preparation time: 10 minutes
Cooking time: 20 minutes
Servings: 4

Ingredients:
- 1 cup white rice
- 2 cups almond milk
- 4 dates, chopped
- 2 tablespoons cinnamon powder
- 2 tablespoons coconut sugar

Directions:
1. In a pot, combine the rice with the milk and the other ingredients, bring to a simmer and cook over medium heat for 20 minutes.
2. Stir the mix again, divide into bowls and serve for breakfast.

Nutrition: calories 516, fat 29, fiber 3.9, carbs 59.4, protein 6.8

Figs, Pear and Pomegranate Yogurt

Preparation time: 10 minutes
Cooking time: 0 minutes
Servings: 4

Ingredients:
- 1 cup figs, halved
- 1 pear, cored and cubed
- ½ cup pomegranate seeds
- ½ cup coconut sugar
- 2 cups non-fat yogurt

Directions:
1. In a bowl, combine the figs with the yogurt and the other ingredients, toss, divide into bowls and serve for breakfast.

Nutrition: calories 223, fat 0.5, fiber 6.1, carbs 52, protein 4.5

Nutmeg Strawberry Porridge

Preparation time: 10 minutes
Cooking time: 20 minutes
Servings: 4

Ingredients:
- 4 cups coconut milk
- 1 cup cornmeal
- 1 teaspoon vanilla extract
- 1 cup strawberries, halved
- ½ teaspoon nutmeg, ground

Directions:
1. Put the milk in a pot, bring to a simmer over medium heat, add the cornmeal and the other ingredients, toss, cook for 20 minutes, and take off the heat.
2. Divide the porridge between plates and serve for breakfast.

Nutrition: calories 678, fat 58.5, fiber 8.3, carbs 39.8, protein 8.2

Creamy Rice and Berries

Preparation time: 10 minutes
Cooking time: 20 minutes
Servings: 4

Ingredients:
- 1 cup brown rice
- 2 cups coconut milk
- 1 tablespoon cinnamon powder
- 1 cup blackberries
- ½ cup coconut cream, unsweetened

Directions:
1. Put the milk in a pot, bring to a simmer over medium heat, add the rice and the other ingredients, cook for 20 minutes, and divide into bowls.
2. Serve warm for breakfast.

Nutrition: calories 469, fat 30.1, fiber 6.5, carbs 47.4, protein 7

Vanilla Coconut Rice

Preparation time: 10 minutes
Cooking time: 20 minutes
Servings: 6

Ingredients:
- 2 cups coconut milk
- 1 cup basmati rice
- 2 tablespoons coconut sugar
- ¾ cup coconut cream
- 1 teaspoon vanilla extract

Directions:
1. In a pot, combine the milk with the rice and the other ingredients, stir, bring to a simmer and cook over medium heat for 20 minutes.
2. Stir the mix again, divide into bowls and serve for breakfast.

Nutrition: calories 462, fat 25.3, fiber 2.2, carbs 55.2, protein 4.8

Coconut Rice and Cherries

Preparation time: 10 minutes
Cooking time: 25 minutes
Servings: 4

Ingredients:
- 1 tablespoon coconut, shredded
- 2 tablespoons coconut sugar
- 1 cup white rice
- 2 cups coconut milk
- ½ teaspoon vanilla extract
- ¼ cup cherries, pitted and halved
- Cooking spray

Directions:
1. Put the milk in a pot, add the sugar and the coconut, stir and bring to a simmer over medium heat.
2. Add the rice and the other ingredients, simmer for 25 minutes stirring often, divide into bowls and serve.

Nutrition: calories 505, fat 29.5, fiber 3.4, carbs 55.7, protein 6.6

Ginger Rice Mix

Preparation time: 10 minutes
Cooking time: 25 minutes
Servings: 4

Ingredients:
- 1 cup white rice
- 2 cups almond milk
- 1 tablespoon ginger, grated
- 3 tablespoons coconut sugar
- 1 teaspoon cinnamon powder

Directions:
1. Put the milk in a pot, bring to a simmer over medium heat, add the rice and the other ingredients, stir, cook for 25 minutes, divide into bowls and serve.

Nutrition: calories 449, fat 29, fiber 3.4, carbs 44.6, protein 6.2

Chili Sausage Casserole

Preparation time: 10 minutes
Cooking time: 35 minutes
Servings: 4

Ingredients:
- 1 pound hash browns
- 4 eggs, whisked
- 1 red onion, chopped
- 1 chili pepper, chopped
- 1 tablespoon olive oil
- 6 ounces low-sodium sausage, chopped
- ¼ teaspoon chili powder
- A pinch of black pepper

Directions:
1. Heat up a pan with the oil over medium heat, add the onion and the sausage, stir and brown for 5 minutes.
2. Add the hash browns and the other ingredients except the eggs and pepper, stir and cook for 5 minutes more.
3. Pour the eggs mixed with the black pepper over the sausage mix, introduce the pan in the oven and bake at 370 degrees F for 25 minutes.
4. Divide the mix between plates and serve fro breakfast,

Nutrition: calories 527, fat 31.3, fiber 3.8, carbs 51.2, protein 13.3

Mushroom Rice Bowls

Preparation time: 10 minutes
Cooking time: 30 minutes
Servings: 4

Ingredients:
- 1 red onion, chopped
- 1 cup white rice
- 2 garlic cloves, minced
- 2 tablespoons olive oil
- 2 cups low-sodium chicken stock
- 1 tablespoon cilantro, chopped
- ½ cup fat-free cheddar cheese, grated
- ½ pound white mushroom, sliced
- Back pepper to the taste

Directions:
1. Heat up a pan with the oil over medium heat, add the onion, garlic and mushrooms, stir and cook for 5-6 minutes.
2. Add the rice and the rest of the ingredients, bring to a simmer and cook over medium heat for 25 minutes stirring often.
3. Divide the rice mix between bowls and serve for breakfast.

Nutrition: calories 314, fat 12.2, fiber 1.8, carbs 42.1, protein 9.5

Tomato and Spinach Eggs

Preparation time: 10 minutes
Cooking time: 20 minutes
Servings: 4

Ingredients:
- ½ cup low-fat milk
- Black pepper to the taste
- 8 eggs, whisked
- 1 cup baby spinach, chopped
- 1 yellow onion, chopped
- 1 tablespoon olive oil
- 1 cup cherry tomatoes, cubed
- ¼ cup fat-free cheddar, grated

Directions:
1. Heat up a pan with the oil over medium heat, add the onion, stir and cook for 2-3 minutes.
2. Add the spinach and tomatoes, stir and cook for 2 minutes more.
3. Add the eggs mixed with the milk and black pepper and toss gently.
4. Sprinkle the cheddar on top, introduce the pan in the oven and cook at 390 degrees F for 15 minutes.
5. Divide between plates and serve.

Nutrition: calories 195, fat 13, fiber 1.3, carbs 6.8, protein 13.7

Sesame Omelet

Preparation time: 5 minutes
Cooking time: 15 minutes
Servings: 4

Ingredients:
- 4 eggs, whisked
- A pinch of black pepper
- 1 tablespoon olive oil
- 1 teaspoon sesame seeds
- 2 scallions, chopped
- 1 teaspoon sweet paprika
- 1 tablespoon cilantro, chopped

Directions:
1. Heat up a pan with the oil over medium heat, add the scallions, stir and sauté for 2 minutes.
2. Add the eggs mixed with the other ingredients, toss a bit, spread the omelet into the pan and cook for 7 minutes.
3. Flip, cook the omelet for 6 minutes more, divide between plates and serve.

Nutrition: calories 101, fat 8.3, fiber 0.5, carbs 1.4, protein 5.9

Zucchini Oatmeal

Preparation time: 5 minutes
Cooking time: 20 minutes
Servings: 4

Ingredients:
- 1 cup steel cut oats
- 3 cups almond milk
- 1 tablespoon fat-free butter
- 2 teaspoons cinnamon powder
- 1 teaspoon pumpkin pie spice
- 1 cup zucchinis, grated

Directions:
1. Heat up a pan with the milk over medium heat, add the oats and the other ingredients, toss, bring to a simmer and cook for 20 minutes, stirring from time to time.
2. Divide the oatmeal into bowls and serve for breakfast.

Nutrition: calories 508, fat 44.5, fiber 6.7, carbs 27.2, protein 7.5

Almonds and Coconut Bowl

Preparation time: 5 minutes
Cooking time: 20 minutes
Servings: 4

Ingredients:
- 2 cups coconut milk
- 1 cup coconut, shredded
- ½ cup maple syrup
- 1 cup raisins
- 1 cup almonds
- ½ teaspoon vanilla extract

Directions:
1. Put the milk in a pot, bring to a simmer over medium heat, add the coconut and the other ingredients, and cook for 20 minutes, stirring from time to time.
2. Divide the mix into bowls and serve warm for breakfast.

Nutrition: calories 697, fat 47.4, fiber 8.8, carbs 70, protein 9.6

Warm Chickpeas Salad

Preparation time: 5 minutes
Cooking time: 15 minutes
Servings: 4

Ingredients:
- 2 garlic cloves, minced
- 2 tomatoes, roughly cubed
- 1 cucumber, roughly cubed
- 2 shallots, chopped
- 2 cups canned chickpeas, no-salt-added, drained
- 1 tablespoon parsley, chopped
- 1/3 cup mint, chopped
- 1 avocado, pitted, peeled and diced
- 2 tablespoons olive oil
- Juice of 1 lime
- Black pepper to the taste

Directions:
1. Heat up a pan with the oil over medium heat, add the garlic and the shallots, stir and cook for 2 minutes.
2. Add the chickpeas and the other ingredients, toss, cook for 13 minutes more, divide into bowls and serve for breakfast.

Nutrition: calories 561, fat 23.1, fiber 22.4, carbs 73.1, protein 21.8

Cocoa Millet Pudding

Preparation time: 10 minutes
Cooking time: 30 minutes
Servings: 4

Ingredients:
- 14 ounces coconut milk
- 1 cup millet
- 1 tablespoon cocoa powder
- ½ teaspoon vanilla extract

Directions:
1. Put the milk in a pot, bring to a simmer over medium heat, add the millet and the other ingredients, and cook for 30 minutes stirring often.
2. Divide into bowls and serve fro breakfast.

Nutrition: calories 422, fat 25.9, fiber 6.8, carbs 42.7, protein 8

Chia Pudding

Preparation time: 15 minutes
Cooking time: 0 minutes
Servings: 4

Ingredients:
- 2 cups almond milk
- ½ cup chia seeds
- 2 tablespoons coconut sugar
- Zest of ½ lemon, grated
- 1 teaspoon vanilla extract
- ½ teaspoon ginger powder

Directions:
1. In a bowl, combine the chia seeds with the milk and the other ingredients, toss and leave aside for 15 minutes before serving.

Nutrition: calories 366, fat 30.8, fiber 5.5, carbs 20.8, protein 4.6

Tapioca Pudding

Preparation time: 2 hours
Cooking time: 0 minutes
Servings: 4

Ingredients:
- ½ cup tapioca pearls
- 2 cups coconut milk, hot
- 4 teaspoons coconut sugar
- ½ teaspoon cinnamon powder

Directions:
1. In a bowl, combine the tapioca with the hot milk and the other ingredients, stir and leave aside for 2 hours before serving.
2. Divide into small bowls and serve for breakfast.

Nutrition: calories 439, fat 28.6, fiber 2.8, carbs 42.5, protein 3.8

Cheddar Hash

Preparation time: 10 minutes
Cooking time: 25 minutes
Servings: 4

Ingredients:
- 1 pound hash browns
- 1 tablespoon avocado oil
- 1/3 cup coconut cream
- 1 yellow onion, chopped
- 1 cup fat-free cheddar cheese, grated
- Black pepper to the taste
- 4 eggs, whisked

Directions:
1. Heat up a pan with the oil over medium heat, add the hash browns and the onion, stir and sauté for 5 minutes.
2. Add the rest of the ingredients except the cheese, toss and cook for 5 minutes more.
3. Sprinkle the cheese on top, introduce the pan in the oven and cook at 390 degrees F for 15 minutes.
4. Divide the mix between plates and serve for breakfast.

Nutrition: calories 539, fat 33.2, fiber 4.8, carbs 44.4, protein 16.8

Snow Peas Salad

Preparation time: 10 minutes
Cooking time: 20 minutes
Servings: 4

Ingredients:
- 3 garlic cloves, minced
- 1 yellow onion, chopped
- 1 tablespoon olive oil
- 1 carrot, chopped
- 1 tablespoon balsamic vinegar
- 2 cups snow peas, halved
- ½ cup veggie stock, no-salt-added
- 2 tablespoons scallions, chopped
- 1 tablespoon cilantro, chopped

Directions:
1. Heat up a pan with the oil over medium heat, add the onion and the garlic, stir and cook for 5 minutes.
2. Add the snow peas and the other ingredients, toss and cook over medium heat for 15 minutes.
3. Divide the mix into bowls and serve warm for breakfast.

Nutrition: calories 89, fat 4.2, fiber 3.3, carbs 11.2, protein 3.3

Quinoa and Chickpeas Mix

Preparation time: 10 minutes
Cooking time: 20 minutes
Servings: 6

Ingredients:
- 1 red onion, chopped
- 1 tablespoon olive oil
- 15 ounces canned chickpeas, no-salt-added and drained
- 14 ounces coconut milk
- ¼ cup quinoa
- 1 tablespoon ginger, grated
- 2 garlic cloves, minced
- 1 tablespoon turmeric powder
- 1 tablespoon cilantro, chopped

Directions:
1. Heat up a pan with the oil over medium heat, add the onion, stir and sauté for 5 minutes.
2. Add the chickpeas, quinoa and the other ingredients, stir, bring to a simmer and cook for 15 minutes.
3. Divide the mix into bowls and serve for breakfast.

Nutrition: calories 472, fat 23, fiber 15.1, carbs 54.6, protein 16.6

Olives and Peppers Salad

Preparation time: 5 minutes
Cooking time: 15 minutes
Servings: 4

Ingredients:
- 1 cup black olives, pitted and halved
- ½ cup green olives, pitted and halved
- 1 tablespoon olive oil
- 2 scallions, chopped
- 1 red bell pepper, cut into strips
- 1 green bell pepper, cut into strips
- Zest of 1 lime, grated
- Juice of 1 lime
- 1 bunch parsley, chopped
- 1 tomato, chopped

Directions:
1. Heat up a pan with the oil over medium heat, add the scallions, stir and sauté for 2 minutes.
2. Add the olives, peppers and the other ingredients, stir and cook for 13 minutes more.
3. Divide into bowls and serve for breakfast.

Nutrition: calories 192, fat 6.7, fiber 3.3, carbs 9.3, protein 3.5

Green Beans and Eggs Mix

Preparation time: 10 minutes
Cooking time: 15 minutes
Servings: 4

Ingredients:
- 1 garlic clove, minced
- 1 red onion, chopped
- 1 tablespoon avocado oil
- 1 pound green beans, trimmed and halved
- 8 eggs, whisked
- 1 tablespoon cilantro, chopped
- A pinch of black pepper

Directions:
1. Heat up a pan with the oil over medium heat, add the onion and the garlic and sauté for 2 minutes.
2. Add the green beans and cook for 2 minutes more.
3. Add the eggs, black pepper and cilantro, toss, spread into the pan and cook for 10 minutes.
4. Divide the mix between plates and serve.

Nutrition: calories 260, fat 12.1, fiber 4.7, carbs 19.4, protein 3.6

Carrot and Eggs Salad

Preparation time: 10 minutes
Cooking time: 0 minutes
Servings: 4

Ingredients:
- 2 carrots, cubed
- 2 green onions, chopped
- 1 bunch of parsley, chopped
- 2 tablespoons olive oil
- 4 eggs, hard boiled, peeled and cubed
- 1 tablespoon balsamic vinegar
- 1 tablespoon chives, chopped
- A pinch of black pepper

Directions:
1. In a bowl, combine the carrots with the eggs and the other ingredients, toss and serve for breakfast.

Nutrition: calories 251, fat 9.6, fiber 4.1, carbs 15.2, protein 3.5

Creamy Berries

Preparation time: 5 minutes
Cooking time: 15 minutes
Servings: 4

Ingredients:
- 3 tablespoons coconut sugar
- 1 cup coconut cream
- 1 cup blueberries
- 1 cup blackberries
- 1 cup strawberries
- 1 teaspoon vanilla extract

Directions:
1. Put the cream in a pot, heat it up over medium heat, add the sugar and the other ingredients, toss, cook for 15 minutes, divide into bowls and serve for breakfast.

Nutrition: calories 460, fat 16.7, fiber 6.5, carbs 40.3, protein 5.7

Apples and Raisins Bowls

Preparation time: 5 minutes
Cooking time: 15 minutes
Servings: 4

Ingredients:
- 1 cup blueberries
- 1 teaspoon cinnamon powder
- 1 and ½ cups almond milk
- ¼ cup raisins
- 2 apples, cored, peeled and cubed
- 1 cup coconut cream

Directions:
1. Put the milk in a pot, bring to a simmer over medium heat, add the berries and the other ingredients, toss, cook for 15 minutes, divide into bowls and serve for breakfast.

Nutrition: calories 482, fat 7.8, fiber 5.6, carbs 15.9, protein 4.9

Ginger Buckwheat Porridge

Preparation time: 10 minutes
Cooking time: 25 minutes
Servings: 4

Ingredients:
- 1 cup buckwheat
- 3 cups coconut milk
- ½ teaspoon vanilla extract
- 1 tablespoon coconut sugar
- 1 teaspoon ginger powder
- 1 teaspoon cinnamon powder

Directions:
1. Put the milk and the sugar in a pot, bring to a simmer over medium heat, add the buckwheat and the other ingredients, cook for 25 minutes, stirring often, divide into bowls and serve for breakfast.

Nutrition: calories 482, fat 14.9, fiber 4.5, carbs 56.3, protein 7.5

Cauliflower and Peppers Salad

Preparation time: 10 minutes
Cooking time: 20 minutes
Servings: 4

Ingredients:
- 1 pound cauliflower florets
- 1 tablespoon olive oil
- 2 spring onions, chopped
- 1 red bell pepper, sliced
- 1 yellow bell pepper, sliced
- 1 green bell pepper, sliced
- 1 tablespoon cilantro, chopped
- A pinch of black pepper

Directions:
1. Heat up a pan with the oil over medium heat, add the spring onions, stir and sauté for 2 minutes.
2. Add the cauliflower and the other ingredients, toss, cook for 16 minutes, divide into bowls and serve for breakfast.

Nutrition: calories 271, fat 11.2 , fiber 3.4, carbs 11.5, protein 4

Chicken and Hash Browns

Preparation time: 10 minutes
Cooking time: 25 minutes
Servings: 4

Ingredients:
- 2 tablespoons olive oil
- 1 yellow onion, chopped
- 2 garlic cloves, minced
- 1 teaspoon Cajun seasoning
- 8 ounces chicken breast, skinless, boneless and ground
- ½ pound hash browns
- 2 tablespoons veggie stock, no-salt-added
- 1 green bell pepper, chopped

Directions:
1. Heat up a pan with the oil over medium heat, add the onion, garlic and the meat and brown for 5 minutes.
2. Add the hash browns and the other ingredients, stir, and cook over medium heat for 20 minutes stirring often.
3. Divide between plates and serve for breakfast.

Nutrition: calories 362, fat 14.3, fiber 6.3, carbs 25.6, protein 6.1

Dash Diet Lunch Recipes

Black Beans Burritos

Preparation time: 5 minutes
Cooking time: 12 minutes
Servings: 4

Ingredients:

- 1 cup canned black beans, no-salt-added, drained and rinsed
- 1 green bell pepper, chopped
- 1 carrots, peeled and grated
- 1 tablespoon olive oil
- 1 red onion, sliced
- ½ cup corn
- 1 cup low-fat cheddar, shredded
- 6 whole wheat tortillas
- 1 cup non-fat yogurt

Directions:

1. Heat up a pan with the oil over medium heat, add the onion and sauté for 2 minutes.
2. Add the beans, carrot, bell pepper and the corn, stir, and cook for 10 minutes more.
3. Arrange the tortillas on a working surface, divide the beans mix on each, also divide the cheese and the yogurt, roll and serve for lunch.

Nutrition: calories 451, fat 7.5, fiber 13.8, carbs 78.2, protein 20.9

Chicken and Mango Mix

Preparation time: 10 minutes
Cooking time: 20 minutes
Servings: 4

Ingredients:
- 2 chicken breasts, skinless, boneless and cubed
- ¼ cup low-sodium chicken stock
- ½ cup celery, chopped
- 1 cup baby spinach
- 1 mango, peeled, and cubed
- 2 spring onions, chopped
- 1 tablespoon olive oil
- 1 teaspoon thyme, dried
- ¼ teaspoon garlic powder
- A pinch of black pepper

Directions:
1. Heat up a pan with the oil over medium-high heat, add the spring onions and the chicken and brown for 5 minutes.
2. Add the celery and the other ingredients except the spinach, toss and cook for 12 minutes more.
3. Add the spinach, toss, cook for 2-3 minutes, divide everything between plates and serve.

Nutrition: calories 221, fat 9.1, fiber 2, carbs 14.1, protein 21.5

Chickpeas Cakes

Preparation time: 10 minutes
Cooking time: 10 minutes
Servings: 4

Ingredients:
- 2 garlic cloves, minced
- 15 ounces canned chickpeas, no-salt-added, drained and rinsed
- 1 teaspoon chili powder
- 1 teaspoon cumin, ground
- 1 egg
- 1 tablespoon olive oil
- 1 tablespoon lime juice
- 1 tablespoon lime zest, grated
- 1 tablespoon cilantro, chopped

Directions:
1. In a blender, combine the chickpeas with the garlic and the other ingredients except the egg and pulse well.
2. Shape medium cakes out of this mix.
3. Heat up a pan with the oil over medium-high heat, add the chickpeas cakes, cook for 5 minutes on each side, divide between plates and serve for lunch with a side salad.

Nutrition: calories 441, fat 11.3, fiber 19, carbs 66.4, protein 22.2

Salsa and Cauliflower Bowls

Preparation time: 10 minutes
Cooking time: 10 minutes
Servings: 4

Ingredients:
- 1 tablespoon avocado oil
- 1 cup red bell peppers, cubed
- 1 pound cauliflower florets
- 1 red onion, chopped
- 3 tablespoons salsa
- 2 tablespoons low-fat cheddar, shredded
- 2 tablespoons coconut cream

Directions:
1. Heat up a pan with the oil over medium-high heat, add the onion and peppers, and sauté for 2 minutes.
2. Add the cauliflower and the other ingredients, toss, cook for 8 minutes more, divide into bowls and serve.

Nutrition: calories 114, fat 5.5, fiber 4.3, carbs 12.7, protein 6.7

Salmon and Spinach Salad

Preparation time: 5 minutes
Cooking time: 0 minutes
Servings: 4

Ingredients:
- 1 cup canned salmon, drained and flaked
- 1 tablespoon lime zest, grated
- 1 tablespoon lime juice
- 3 tablespoons fat-free yogurt
- 1 cup baby spinach
- 1 teaspoon capers, drained and chopped
- 1 red onion, chopped
- A pinch of black pepper
- 1 tablespoon chives, chopped

Directions:
1. In a bowl, combine the salmon with lime zest, lime juice and the other ingredients, toss and serve cold for lunch.

Nutrition: calories 61, fat 1.9, fiber 1, carbs 5, protein 6.8

Chicken and Kale Mix

Preparation time: 10 minutes
Cooking time: 20 minutes
Servings: 4

Ingredients:
- 1 tablespoon olive oil
- 1 pound chicken breast, skinless, boneless and cubed
- ½ pound kale, torn
- 2 cherry tomatoes, halved
- 1 yellow onion, chopped
- ½ cup low-sodium chicken stock
- ¼ cup low-fat mozzarella, shredded

Directions:
1. Heat up a pan with the oil over medium heat, add the chicken and the onion and brown for 5 minutes.
2. Add the kale and the other ingredients except the mozzarella, toss, and cook for 12 minutes more.
3. Sprinkle the cheese on top, cook the mix for 2-3 minutes, divide between plates and serve for lunch.

Nutrition: calories 231, fat 6.5, fiber 2.7, carbs 11.4, protein 30.9

Salmon and Arugula Salad

Preparation time: 10 minutes
Cooking time: 0 minutes
Servings: 4

Ingredients:
- 6 ounces canned salmon, drained and cubed
- 1 tablespoon balsamic vinegar
- 1 tablespoon olive oil
- 2 shallots, chopped
- ½ cup black olives, pitted and halved
- 2 cups baby arugula
- A pinch of black pepper

Directions:
1. In a bowl, combine the salmon with the shallots and the other ingredients, toss and keep in the fridge for 10 minutes before serving for lunch.

Nutrition: calories 113, fat 8, fiber 0.7, carbs 2.3, protein 8.8

Shrimp and Veggies Salad

Preparation time: 5 minutes
Cooking time: 10 minutes
Servings: 4

Ingredients:
- 1 tablespoon olive oil
- 1 pound shrimp, peeled and deveined
- 1 tablespoon basil pesto
- 1 cup baby arugula
- 1 yellow onion, chopped
- 1 cucumber, sliced
- 1 cup carrots, shredded
- 1 tablespoon cilantro, chopped

Directions:
1. Heat up a pan with the oil over medium heat, add the onion and carrots, stir and cook for 3 minutes.
2. Add the shrimp and the other ingredients, toss, cook for 7 minutes more, divide into bowls and serve.

Nutrition: calories 200, fat 5.6, fiber 1.8, carbs 9.9, protein 27

Turkey and Peppers Wraps

Preparation time: 10 minutes
Cooking time: 3 minutes
Servings: 2

Ingredients:
- 2 whole wheat tortillas
- 2 teaspoons mustard
- 2 teaspoons mayonnaise
- 1 turkey breast, skinless, boneless and cut into strips
- 1 tablespoons olive oil
- 1 red onion, chopped
- 1 red bell peppers, cut into strips
- 1 green bell pepper, cut into strips
- ¼ cup low-fat mozzarella, shredded

Directions:
1. Heat up a pan with the oil over medium heat, add the meat and the onion and brown for 5 minutes
2. Add the peppers, toss and cook for 10 minutes more.
3. Arrange the tortillas on a working surface, divide the turkey mix on each, also divide the mayo, mustard and the cheese, wrap and serve for lunch.

Nutrition: calories 342, fat 11.6, fiber 7.7, carbs 39.5, protein 21.9

Green Beans Soup

Preparation time: 5 minutes
Cooking time: 25 minutes
Servings: 4

Ingredients:
- 2 teaspoons olive oil
- 2 garlic cloves, minced
- 1 pound green beans, trimmed and halved
- 1 yellow onion, chopped
- 2 tomatoes, cubed
- 1 teaspoon sweet paprika
- 1 quart low-sodium chicken stock
- 2 tablespoons parsley, chopped

Directions:
1. Heat up a pot with the oil over medium-high heat, add the garlic and the onion, stir and sauté for 5 minutes.
2. Add the green beans and the other ingredients except the parsley, stir, bring to a simmer and cook for 20 minutes.
3. Add the parsley, stir, divide the soup into bowls and serve.

Nutrition: calories 87, fat 2.7, fiber 5.5, carbs 14, protein 4.1

Avocado, Spinach and Olives Salad

Preparation time: 5 minutes
Cooking time: 0 minutes
Servings: 4

Ingredients:
- 2 tablespoon balsamic vinegar
- 2 tablespoons mint, chopped
- A pinch of black pepper
- 1 avocado, peeled, pitted and sliced
- 4 cups baby spinach
- 1 cup black olives, pitted and halved
- 1 cucumber, sliced
- 1 tablespoon olive oil

Directions:
1. In a salad bowl, combine the avocado with the spinach and the other ingredients, toss and serve for lunch.

Nutrition: calories 192, fat 17.1, fiber 5.7, carbs 10.6, protein 2.7

Beef and Zucchini Pan

Preparation time: 5 minutes
Cooking time: 20 minutes
Servings: 4

Ingredients:
- 1 pound beef, ground
- ½ cup yellow onion, chopped
- 1 tablespoon olive oil
- 1 cup zucchini, cubed
- 2 garlic cloves, minced
- 14 ounces canned tomatoes, no-salt-added, chopped
- 1 teaspoon Italian seasoning
- ¼ cup low-fat parmesan, shredded
- 1 tablespoon chives, chopped
- 1 tablespoon cilantro, chopped

Directions:
1. Heat up a pan with the oil over medium heat, add the garlic, onion and the beef and brown for 5 minutes.
2. Add the rest of the ingredients, toss, cook for 15 minutes more, divide into bowls and serve for lunch.

Nutrition: calories 276, fat 11.3, fiber 1.9, carbs 6.8, protein 36

Thyme Beef and Potatoes Mix

Preparation time: 10 minutes
Cooking time: 25 minutes
Servings: 4

Ingredients:

- ½ pound beef, ground
- 3 tablespoons olive oil
- 1 and ¾ pounds red potatoes, peeled and roughly cubed
- 1 yellow onion, chopped
- 2 teaspoons thyme, dried
- 1 cup canned tomatoes, no-salt-added, and chopped
- A pinch of black pepper

Directions:

1. Heat up a pan with the oil over medium-high heat, add the onion and the beef, stir and brown for 5 minutes.
2. Add the potatoes and the rest of the ingredients, toss, bring to a simmer, cook for 20 minutes more, divide into bowls and serve for lunch.

Nutrition: calories 216, fat 14.5, fiber 5.2, carbs 40.7, protein 22.2

Pork and Carrots Soup

Preparation time: 10 minutes
Cooking time: 25 minutes
Servings: 4

Ingredients:
- 1 tablespoon olive oil
- 1 red onion, chopped
- 1 pound pork stew meat, cubed
- 1 quart low-sodium beef stock
- 1 pound carrots, sliced
- 1 cup tomato puree
- 1 tablespoon cilantro, chopped

Directions:
1. Heat up a pot with the oil over medium-high heat, add the onion and the meat and brown for 5 minutes.
2. Add the rest of the ingredients except the cilantro, bring to a simmer, reduce heat to medium, and boil the soup for 20 minutes.
3. Ladle into bowls and serve for lunch with the cilantro sprinkled on top.

Nutrition: calories 354, fat 14.6, fiber 4.6, carbs 19.3, protein 36

Shrimp and Strawberry Salad

Preparation time: 5 minutes
Cooking time: 7 minutes
Servings: 4

Ingredients:
- 1 cup corn
- 1 endive, shredded
- 1 cup baby spinach
- 1 pound shrimp, peeled and deveined
- 2 garlic cloves, minced
- 1 tablespoon lime juice
- 2 cups strawberries, halved
- 2 tablespoons olive oil
- 2 tablespoons balsamic vinegar
- 1 tablespoon cilantro, chopped

Directions:
1. Heat up a pan with the oil over medium-high heat, add the garlic and brown for 1 minute.
Add the shrimp and lime juice, toss and cook for 3 minutes on each side.
2. In a salad bowl, combine the shrimp with the corn, endive and the other ingredients, toss and serve for lunch.

Nutrition: calories 260, fat 9.7, fiber 2.9, carbs 16.5, protein 28

Shrimp and Green Beans Salad

Preparation time: 5 minutes
Cooking time: 10 minutes
Servings: 4

Ingredients:
- 1 pound green beans, trimmed and halved
- 2 tablespoons olive oil
- 2 pounds shrimp, peeled and deveined
- 1 tablespoon lemon juice
- 2 cups cherry tomatoes, halved
- ¼ cup raspberry vinegar
- A pinch of black pepper

Directions:
1. Heat up a pan with the oil over medium-high heat, add the shrimp, toss and cook for 2 minutes.
2. Add the green beans and the other ingredients, toss, cook for 8 minutes more, divide into bowls and serve for lunch.

Nutrition: calories 385, fat 11.2, fiber 5, carbs 15.3, protein 54.5

Fish Tacos

Preparation time: 10 minutes
Cooking time: 10 minutes
Servings: 2

Ingredients:
- 4 whole wheat taco shells
- 1 tablespoon light mayonnaise
- 1 tablespoon salsa
- 1 tablespoon low-fat mozzarella, shredded
- 1 tablespoon olive oil
- 1 red onion, chopped
- 1 tablespoon cilantro, chopped
- 2 cod fillets, boneless, skinless and cubed
- 1 tablespoon tomato puree

Directions:
1. Heat up a pan with the oil over medium heat, add the onion, stir and cook for 2 minutes.
2. Add the fish and tomato puree, toss gently and cook for 5 minutes more.
3. Spoon this into the taco shells, also divide the mayo, salsa and the cheese and serve for lunch.

Nutrition: calories 466, fat 14.5, fiber 8, carbs 56.6, protein 32.9

Zucchini Cakes

Preparation time: 10 minutes
Cooking time: 10 minutes
Servings: 4

Ingredients:
- 1 yellow onion, chopped
- 2 zucchinis, grated
- 2 tablespoons almond flour
- 1 egg, whisked
- 1 garlic clove, minced
- A pinch of black pepper
- 1/3 cup carrot, shredded
- 1/3 cup low-fat cheddar, grated
- 1 tablespoon cilantro, chopped
- 1 teaspoon lemon zest, grated
- 2 tablespoons olive oil

Directions:
1. In a bowl, combine the zucchinis with the garlic, onion and the other ingredients except the oil, stir well and shape medium cakes out of this mix.
2. Heat up a pan with the oil over medium-high heat, add the zucchini cakes, cook for 5 minutes on each side, divide between plates and serve with a side salad.

Nutrition: calories 271, fat 8.7, fiber 4, carbs 14.3, protein 4.6

Chickpeas and Tomatoes Stew

Preparation time: 10 minutes
Cooking time: 20 minutes
Servings: 4

Ingredients:
- 1 tablespoon olive oil
- 1 yellow onion, chopped
- 2 teaspoons chili powder
- 14 ounces canned chickpeas, no-salt-added, drained and rinsed
- 14 ounces canned tomatoes, no-salt-added, cubed
- 1 cup low-sodium chicken stock
- 1 tablespoon cilantro, chopped
- A pinch of black pepper

Directions:
1. Heat up a pot with the oil over medium-high heat, add the onion and chili powder, stir and cook for 5 minutes.
2. Add the chickpeas and the other ingredients, toss, cook for 15 minutes over medium heat, divide into bowls and serve for lunch.

Nutrition: calories 299, fat 13.2, fiber 4.7, carbs 17.2, protein 8.1

Chicken, Tomato and Spinach Salad

Preparation time: 10 minutes
Cooking time: 0 minutes
Servings: 4

Ingredients:
- 1 tablespoon olive oil
- A pinch of black pepper
- 2 rotisserie chicken, skinless, boneless, shredded
- 1 pound cherry tomatoes, halved
- 1 red onion, chopped
- 4 cups baby spinach
- ¼ cup walnuts, chopped
- ½ teaspoon lemon zest, grated
- 2 tablespoons lemon juice

Directions:
1. In a salad bowl, combine the chicken with the tomato and the other ingredients, toss and serve for lunch.

Nutrition: calories 349, fat 8.3, fiber 5.6, carbs 16.9, protein 22.8

Asparagus and Peppers Bowls

Preparation time: 10 minutes
Cooking time: 20 minutes
Servings: 4

Ingredients:
- 3 garlic cloves, minced
- 2 tablespoons olive oil
- 1 red onion, chopped
- 3 carrots, sliced
- ½ cup low-sodium chicken stock
- 2 cups baby spinach
- 1 pound asparagus, trimmed and halved
- 1 red bell pepper, cut into strips
- 1 yellow bell pepper, cut into strips
- 1 green bell pepper, cut into strips
- A pinch of black pepper

Directions:
1. Heat up a pan with the oil over medium-high heat, add the onion and the garlic, stir and sauté for 2 minutes.
2. Add the asparagus and the other ingredients except the spinach, toss, and cook for 15 minutes.
3. Add the spinach, cook everything for 3 minutes more, divide into bowls and serve for lunch.

Nutrition: calories 221, fat 11.2, fiber 3.4, carbs 14.3, protein 5.9

Hot Beef Stew

Preparation time: 10 minutes
Cooking time: 1 hour and 20 minutes

Servings: 4

Ingredients:
- 1 pound beef stew meat, cubed
- 1 cup no-salt-added tomato sauce
- 1 cup low-sodium beef stock
- 1 tablespoon olive oil
- 1 yellow onion, chopped
- ¼ teaspoon hot sauce
- 1 teaspoon onion powder
- 1 teaspoon garlic powder
- 1 tablespoon cilantro, chopped

Directions:
1. Heat up a pot with the oil over medium-high heat, add the meat and the onion, stir and brown for 5 minutes.
2. Add the tomato sauce and the rest of the ingredients, bring to a simmer and cook over medium heat for 1 hour and 15 minutes.
3. Divide into bowls and serve for lunch.

Nutrition: calories 487, fat 15.3, fiber 5.8, carbs 56.3, protein 15

Pork Chops with Mushrooms

Preparation time: 5 minutes
Cooking time: 8 hours and 10 minutes

Servings: 4

Ingredients:
- 4 pork chops
- 1 tablespoon olive oil
- 2 shallots, chopped
- 1 pound white mushrooms, sliced
- ½ cup low-sodium beef stock
- 1 tablespoon rosemary, chopped
- ¼ teaspoon garlic powder
- 1 teaspoon sweet paprika

Directions:
1. Heat up a pan with the oil over medium-high heat, add the pork chops and the shallots, toss, brown for 10 minutes and transfer to a slow cooker.
2. Add the rest of the ingredients, put the lid on and cook on Low for 8 hours.
3. Divide the pork chops and mushrooms between plates and serve for lunch.

Nutrition: calories 349, fat 24, fiber 5.6, carbs 46.3, protein 17.5

Coriander Shrimp Salad

Preparation time: 10 minutes
Cooking time: 8 minutes
Servings: 4

Ingredients:
- 1 tablespoon olive oil
- 1 red onion, sliced
- 1 pound shrimp, peeled and deveined
- 2 cups baby arugula
- 1 tablespoon balsamic vinegar
- 1 tablespoon lemon juice
- 1 tablespoon coriander, chopped
- A pinch of black pepper

Directions:
1. Heat up a pan with the oil over medium heat, add the onion, stir and sauté for 2 minutes.
2. Add the shrimp and the other ingredients, toss, cook for 6 minutes, divide into bowls and serve for lunch.

Nutrition: calories 341, fat 11.5, fiber 3.8, carbs 17.3, protein 14.3

Eggplant Stew

Preparation time: 5 minutes
Cooking time: 20 minutes
Servings: 4

Ingredients:
- 1 pound eggplants, roughly cubed
- 2 garlic cloves, minced
- 2 tablespoons olive oil
- 1 yellow onion, chopped
- 1 teaspoon sweet paprika
- ½ cup cilantro, chopped
- 14 ounces low-sodium canned tomatoes, chopped
- 1 tablespoon cilantro, chopped

Directions:
1. Heat up a pan with the oil over medium-high heat, add the onion and the garlic and sauté for 2 minutes.
2. Add the eggplant and the other ingredients except the cilantro, bring to a simmer and cook for 18 minutes.
3. Divide into bowls and serve with the cilantro sprinkled on top.

Nutrition: calories 343, fat 12.3, fiber 3.7, carbs 16.56, protein 7.2

Beef and Peas Mix

Preparation time: 10 minutes
Cooking time: 30 minutes
Servings: 4

Ingredients:
- 1 and ¼ cups low-sodium beef stock
- 1 yellow onion, chopped
- 1 tablespoon olive oil
- 2 cups peas
- 1 pound beef stew meat, cubed
- 1 cup canned tomatoes, no-salt-added and chopped
- 1 cup scallions, chopped
- ¼ cup parsley, chopped
- Black pepper to the taste

Directions:
1. Heat up a pot with the oil over medium-high heat, add the onion and the meat and brown for 5 minutes.
2. Add the peas and the other ingredients, stir, bring to a simmer and cook over medium heat for 25 minutes more.
3. Divide the mix into bowls and serve for lunch.

Nutrition: calories 487, fat 15.4, fiber 4.6, carbs 44.6, protein 17.8

Turkey Stew

Preparation time: 5 minutes
Cooking time: 30 minutes
Servings: 4

Ingredients:
- 2 tablespoons olive oil
- 1 turkey breast, skinless, boneless and cubed
- 1 cup low-sodium beef stock
- 1 cup tomato puree
- ¼ teaspoon lime zest, grated
- 1 yellow onion, chopped
- 1 tablespoon sweet paprika
- 1 tablespoon cilantro, chopped
- 2 tablespoons lime juice
- ¼ teaspoon ginger, grated

Directions:
1. Heat up a pot with the oil over medium-high heat, add the onion and the meat and brown for 5 minutes.
2. Add the stock and the other ingredients, bring to a simmer and cook over medium heat for 25 minutes.
3. Divide the mix into bowls and serve for lunch.

Nutrition: calories 150, fat 8.1, fiber 2.7, carbs 12, protein 9.5

Beef Salad

Preparation time: 10 minutes
Cooking time: 30 minutes
Servings: 4

Ingredients:
- 1 pound beef stew meat, cut into strips
- 1 tablespoon sage, chopped
- 1 tablespoon olive oil
- A pinch of black pepper
- ½ teaspoon cumin, ground
- 2 cups cherry tomatoes, cubed
- 1 avocado, peeled, pitted and cubed
- 1 cup canned black beans, no-salt-added, drained and rinsed
- ½ cup green onions, chopped
- 2 tablespoons lime juice
- 2 tablespoons balsamic vinegar
- 2 tablespoons cilantro, chopped

Directions:
1. Heat up a pan with the oil over medium-high heat, add the meat and brown for 5 minutes.
2. Add the sage, black pepper and the cumin, toss and cook for 5 minutes more.
3. Add the rest of the ingredients, toss, reduce heat to medium and cook the mix for 20 minutes.
4. Divide the salad into bowls and serve for lunch.

Nutrition: calories 536, fat 21.4, fiber 12.5, carbs 40.4, protein 47

Squash Stew

Preparation time: 10 minutes
Cooking time: 20 minutes
Servings: 4

Ingredients:
- 1 pound squash, peeled and roughly cubed
- 1 cup low-sodium chicken stock
- 1 cup canned tomatoes, no-salt-added, crushed
- 1 tablespoon olive oil
- 1 red onion, chopped
- 2 orange sweet peppers, chopped
- ½ cup quinoa
- ½ tablespoon chives, chopped

Directions:
1. Heat up a pot with the oil over medium heat, add the onion, stir and sauté for 2 minutes.
2. Add the squash and the other ingredients, bring to a simmer, and cook for 15 minutes.
3. Stir the stew, divide into bowls and serve for lunch.

Nutrition: calories 166, fat 5.3, fiber 4.7, carbs 26.3, protein 5.9

Cabbage and Beef Mix

Preparation time: 10 minutes
Cooking time: 20 minutes
Servings: 4

Ingredients:
- 1 green cabbage head, shredded
- ¼ cup low-sodium beef stock
- 2 tomatoes, cubed
- 2 yellow onions, chopped
- ¾ cup red bell peppers, chopped
- 1 tablespoon olive oil
- 1 pound beef, ground
- ¼ cup cilantro, chopped
- ¼ cup green onions, chopped
- ¼ teaspoon red pepper, crushed

Directions:
1. Heat up a pan with the oil over medium heat, add the meat and the onions, stir and brown for 5 minutes.
2. Add the cabbage and the other ingredients, toss, cook for 15 minutes, divide into bowls and serve for lunch.

Nutrition: calories 328, fat 11, fiber 6.9, carbs 20.1, protein 38.3

Pork and Green Beans Stew

Preparation time: 5 minutes
Cooking time: 8 hours and 10 minutes

Servings: 4

Ingredients:
- 1 pound pork stew meat, cubed
- 1 tablespoon olive oil
- ½ pound green beans, trimmed and halved
- 2 yellow onions, chopped
- 2 garlic cloves, minced
- 2 cups low-sodium beef stock
- 8 ounces tomato sauce
- A pinch of black pepper
- A pinch of allspice, ground
- 1 tablespoon rosemary, chopped

Directions:
1. Heat up a pan with the oil over medium-high heat, add the meat, garlic and onion, stir and brown for 10 minutes.
2. Transfer this to a slow cooker, add the other ingredients as well, put the lid on and cook on Low for 8 hours.
3. Divide the stew into bowls and serve.

Nutrition: calories 334, fat 14.8, fiber 4.4, carbs 13.3, protein 36.7

Zucchini Cream Soup

Preparation time: 10 minutes
Cooking time: 20 minutes
Servings: 4

Ingredients:
- 1 tablespoon olive oil
- 1 yellow onion, chopped
- 1 teaspoon ginger, grated
- 1 pound zucchinis, chopped
- 32 ounces low-sodium chicken stock
- 1 cup coconut cream
- 1 tablespoon dill, chopped

Directions:
1. Heat up a pot with the oil over medium heat, add the onion and ginger, stir and cook for 5 minutes.
2. Add the zucchinis and the other ingredients, bring to a simmer and cook over medium heat for 15 minutes.
3. Blend using an immersion blender, divide into bowls and serve.

Nutrition: calories 293, fat 12.3, fiber 2.7, carbs 11.2, protein 6.4

Shrimp and Grapes Salad

Preparation time: 5 minutes
Cooking time: 0 minutes
Servings: 4

Ingredients:
- 2 tablespoons low-fat mayonnaise
- 2 teaspoons chili powder
- A pinch of black pepper
- 1 pound shrimp, cooked, peeled and deveined
- 1 cup red grapes, halved
- ½ cup scallions, chopped
- ¼ cup walnuts, chopped
- 1 tablespoon cilantro, chopped

Directions:
1. In a salad bowl, combine shrimp with the chili powder and the other ingredients, toss and serve fro lunch.

Nutrition: calories 298, fat 12.3, fiber 2.6, carbs 16.2, protein 7.8

Turmeric Carrot Cream

Preparation time: 5 minutes
Cooking time: 25 minutes
Servings: 4

Ingredients:
- 2 tablespoons olive oil
- 1 yellow onion, chopped
- 1 pound carrots, peeled and chopped
- 1 teaspoon turmeric powder
- 4 celery stalks, chopped
- 5 cups low-sodium chicken stock
- A pinch of black pepper
- 1 tablespoon cilantro, chopped

Directions:
1. Heat up a pot with the oil over medium heat, add the onion, stir and sauté for 2 minutes.
2. Add the carrots and the other ingredients, bring to a simmer and cook over medium heat for 20 minutes.
3. Blend the soup using an immersion blender, ladle into bowls and serve.

Nutrition: calories 221, fat 9.6, fiber 4.7, carbs 16, protein 4.8

Beef and Black Beans Soup

Preparation time: 10 minutes
Cooking time: 1 hour and 40 minutes

Servings: 4

Ingredients:
- 1 cup canned black beans, no-salt-added and drained
- 7 cups low-sodium beef stock
- 1 green bell pepper, chopped
- 1 tablespoon olive oil
- 1 pound beef stew meat, cubed
- 1 yellow onion, chopped
- 3 garlic cloves, minced
- 1 chili pepper, chopped
- 1 potato, cubed
- A pinch of black pepper
- 1 tablespoon cilantro, chopped

Directions:
1. Heat up a pot with the oil over medium heat, add the onion, garlic and the meat, and brown for 5 minutes.
2. Add the beans and the rest of the ingredients except the cilantro, bring to a simmer and cook over medium heat for 1 hour and 35 minutes.
3. Add the cilantro, ladle the soup into bowls and serve.

Nutrition: calories 421, fat 17.3, fiber 3.8, carbs 18.8, protein 23.5

Salmon and Shrimp Bowls

Preparation time: 10 minutes
Cooking time: 13 minutes
Servings: 4

Ingredients:
- ½ pound smoked salmon, boneless, skinless and cubed
- ½ pound shrimp, peeled and deveined
- 1 tablespoon olive oil
- 1 red onion, chopped
- ¼ cup tomatoes, cubed
- ½ cup mild salsa
- 2 tablespoons cilantro, chopped

Directions:
1. Heat up a pan with the oil over medium-high heat, add the salmon, toss and cook for 5 minutes.
2. Add the onion, shrimp and the other ingredients, cook for 7 minutes more, divide into bowls and serve.

Nutrition: calories 251, fat 11.4, fiber 3.7, carbs 12.3, protein 7.1

Chicken and Garlic Sauce

Preparation time: 5 minutes
Cooking time: 20 minutes
Servings: 4

Ingredients:
- 1 tablespoon olive oil
- 1 yellow onion, chopped
- A pinch of black pepper
- 1 pound chicken breasts, skinless, boneless and cubed
- 4 garlic cloves, minced
- 1 cup low-sodium chicken stock
- 2 cups coconut cream
- 1 tablespoon basil, chopped
- 1 tablespoon chives, chopped

Directions:
1. Heat up a pan with the oil over medium-high heat, add the garlic, onion and the meat, toss and brown for 5 minutes.
2. Add the stock and the rest of the ingredients, bring to a simmer and cook over medium heat for 15 minutes.
3. Divide the mix between plates and serve.

Nutrition: calories 451, fat 16.6, fiber 9, carbs 34.4, protein 34.5

Turmeric Chicken and Eggplant Stew

Preparation time: 5 minutes
Cooking time: 20 minutes
Servings: 4

Ingredients:
- 1 pound chicken breasts, skinless, boneless and cubed
- 2 shallots, chopped
- 1 tablespoon olive oil
- 1 eggplant, cubed
- 1 cup canned tomatoes, no-salt-added and crushed
- 1 tablespoon lime juice
- A pinch of black pepper
- ¼ teaspoon ginger, ground
- 1 tablespoon cilantro, chopped

Directions:
1. Heat up a pot with the oil over medium heat, add the shallots and the chicken and brown for 5 minutes.
2. Add the rest of the ingredients, bring to a simmer and cook over medium heat for 15 minutes more.
3. Divide into bowls and serve for lunch.

Nutrition: calories 441, fat 14.6, fiber 4.9, carbs 44.4, protein 16.9

Chicken and Endives Mix

Preparation time: 5 minutes
Cooking time: 20 minutes
Servings: 4

Ingredients:
- 1 pound chicken thighs, boneless, skinless and cubed
- 2 endives, shredded
- 1 cup low-sodium chicken stock
- 1 tablespoon olive oil
- 1 yellow onion, chopped
- 1 carrot, sliced
- 2 garlic cloves, minced
- 8 ounces canned tomatoes, no-salt-added, chopped
- 1 tablespoon chives, chopped

Directions:
1. Heat up a pan with the oil over medium-high heat, add the onion and garlic and sauté for 5 minutes.
2. Add the chicken and brown for 5 minutes more.
3. Add the rest of the ingredients, bring to a simmer, cook for 10 minutes more, divide between plates and serve.

Nutrition: calories 411, fat 16.7, fiber 5.9, carbs 54.5, protein 24

Turkey Soup

Preparation time: 10 minutes
Cooking time: 40 minutes
Servings: 4

Ingredients:
- 1 turkey breast, skinless, boneless, cubed
- 1 tablespoon tomato sauce, no-salt-added
- 1 tablespoon olive oil
- 2 yellow onions, chopped
- 1 quart low-sodium chicken stock
- 1 tablespoon oregano, chopped
- 2 carrots, sliced
- 3 garlic cloves, minced
- A pinch of black pepper

Directions:
1. Heat up a pot with the oil over medium heat, add the onions and the garlic and sauté for 5 minutes.
2. Add the meat and brown it for 5 minutes more.
3. Add the rest of the ingredients, bring to a simmer and cook over medium heat for 30 minutes.
4. Ladle the soup into bowls and serve.

Nutrition: calories 321, fat 14.5, fiber 11.3, carbs 33.7, protein 16

Shrimp and Pineapple mix

Preparation time: 10 minutes
Cooking time: 10 minutes
Servings: 4

Ingredients:
- 1 tablespoon olive oil
- 1 pound shrimp, peeled and deveined
- 1 cup pineapple, peeled and cubed
- Juice of 1 lemon
- A bunch of parsley, chopped

Directions:
1. Heat up a pan with the oil over medium heat, add the shrimp and cook for 3 minutes on each side.
2. Add the rest of the ingredients, cook everything for 4 minutes more, divide into bowls and serve.

Nutrition: calories 254, fat 13.3, fiber 6, carbs 14.9, protein 11

Salmon and Green Olives

Preparation time: 10 minutes
Cooking time: 20 minutes
Servings: 4

Ingredients:
- 1 yellow onion, chopped
- 1 cup green olives, pitted and halved
- 1 teaspoon chili powder
- Black pepper to the taste
- 2 tablespoons olive oil
- ¼ cup low-sodium veggie stock
- 4 salmon fillets, skinless and boneless
- 2 tablespoons chives, chopped

Directions:
1. Heat up a pan with the oil over medium-high heat, add the onion and sauté for 3 minutes.
2. Add the salmon and cook for 5 minutes on each side. Add the rest of the ingredients, cook the mix for 5 minutes more, divide between plates and serve.

Nutrition: calories 221, fat 12.1, fiber 5.4, carbs 8.5, protein 11.2

Salmon and Fennel

Preparation time: 5 minutes
Cooking time: 15 minutes
Servings: 4

Ingredients:
- 4 medium salmon fillets, skinless and boneless
- 1 fennel bulb, chopped
- ½ cup low-sodium veggie stock
- 2 tablespoons olive oil
- Black pepper to the taste
- ¼ cup low-sodium veggie stock
- 1 tablespoon lemon juice
- 1 tablespoon cilantro, chopped

Directions:
1. Heat up a pan with the oil over medium heat, add the fennel and cook for 3 minutes.
2. Add the fish and brown it for 4 minutes on each side.
3. Add the rest of the ingredients, cook everything for 4 minutes more, divide between plates and serve.

Nutrition: calories 252, fat 9.3, fiber 4.2, carbs 12.3, protein 9

Cod and Asparagus

Preparation time: 10 minutes
Cooking time: 14 minutes
Servings: 4

Ingredients:
- 1 tablespoon olive oil
- 1 red onion, chopped
- 1 pound cod fillets, boneless
- 1 bunch asparagus, trimmed
- Black pepper to the taste
- 1 cup coconut cream
- 1 tablespoon chives, chopped

Directions:
1. Heat up a pan with the oil over medium heat, add the onion and the cod and cook it for 3 minutes on each side.
2. Add the rest of the ingredients, cook everything for 8 minutes more, divide between plates and serve.

Nutrition: calories 254, fat 12.1, fiber 5.4, carbs 4.2, protein 13.5

Spiced Shrimp

Preparation time: 5 minutes
Cooking time: 8 minutes
Servings: 4

Ingredients:
- 1 teaspoon garlic powder
- 1 teaspoon smoked paprika
- 1 teaspoon cumin, ground
- 1 teaspoon allspice, ground
- 2 tablespoons olive oil
- 2 pounds shrimp, peeled and deveined
- 1 tablespoon chives, chopped

Directions:
1. Heat up a pan with the oil over medium heat, add the shrimp, garlic powder and the other ingredients, cook for 4 minutes on each side, divide into bowls and serve.

Nutrition: calories 212, fat 9.6, fiber 5.3, carbs 12.7, protein 15.4

Sea Bass and Tomatoes

Preparation time: 10 minutes
Cooking time: 30 minutes
Servings: 4

Ingredients:
- 2 tablespoons olive oil
- 2 pounds sea bass fillets, skinless and boneless
- Black pepper to the taste
- 2 cups cherry tomatoes, halved
- 1 tablespoon chives, chopped
- 1 tablespoon lemon zest, grated
- ¼ cup lemon juice

Directions:
1. Grease a roasting pan with the oil and arrange the fish inside.
2. Add the tomatoes and the other ingredients, introduce the pan in the oven and bake at 380 degrees F for 30 minutes.
3. Divide everything between plates and serve.

Nutrition: calories 272, fat 6.9, fiber 6.2, carbs 18.4, protein 9

Shrimp and Beans

Preparation time: 10 minutes
Cooking time: 12 minutes
Servings: 4

Ingredients:
- 1 pound shrimp, deveined and peeled
- 1 tablespoon olive oil
- Juice of 1 lime
- 1 cup canned black beans, no-salt-added, drained
- 1 shallot, chopped
- 1 tablespoon oregano, chopped
- 2 garlic cloves, chopped
- Black pepper to the taste

Directions:
1. Heat up a pan with the oil over medium-high heat, add the shallot and the garlic, stir and cook for 3 minutes.
2. Add the shrimp and cook for 2 minutes on each side.
3. Add the beans and the other ingredients, cook everything over medium heat for 5 minutes more, divide into bowls and serve.

Nutrition: calories 253, fat 11.6, fiber 6, carbs 14.5, protein 13.5

Shrimp and Horseradish Mix

Preparation time: 5 minutes
Cooking time: 8 minutes
Servings: 4

Ingredients:
- 1 pound shrimp, peeled and deveined
- 2 shallots, chopped
- 1 tablespoon olive oil
- 1 tablespoon chives, chopped
- 2 teaspoons prepared horseradish
- ¼ cup coconut cream
- Black pepper to the taste

Directions:
4 Heat up a pan with the oil over medium heat, add the shallots and the horseradish, stir and sauté for 2 minutes.
5 Add the shrimp and the other ingredients, toss, cook for 6 minutes more, divide between plates and serve.

Nutrition: calories 233, fat 6, fiber 5, carbs 11.9, protein 5.4

Shrimp and Tarragon Salad

Preparation time: 4 minutes
Cooking time: 0 minutes
Servings: 4

Ingredients:
- 1 pound shrimp, cooked, peeled and deveined
- 1 tablespoon tarragon, chopped
- 1 tablespoon capers, drained
- 2 tablespoons olive oil
- Black pepper to the taste
- 2 cups baby spinach
- 1 tablespoon balsamic vinegar
- 1 small red onion, sliced
- 2 tablespoons lemon juice

Directions:
4 In a bowl, combine the shrimp with the tarragon and the other ingredients, toss and serve.

Nutrition: calories 258, fat 12.4, fiber 6, carbs 6.7, protein 13.3

Parmesan Cod Mix

Preparation time: 10 minutes
Cooking time: 20 minutes
Servings: 4

Ingredients:
- 4 cod fillets, boneless
- ½ cup low-fat parmesan cheese, shredded
- 3 garlic cloves, minced
- 1 tablespoon olive oil
- 1 tablespoon lemon juice
- ½ cup green onion, chopped

Directions:
1. Heat up a pan with the oil over medium heat, add the garlic and the green onions, toss and sauté for 5 minutes.
2. Add the fish and cook it for 4 minutes on each side.
3. Add the lemon juice, sprinkle the parmesan on top, cook everything for 2 minutes more, divide between plates and serve.

Nutrition: calories 275, fat 22.1, fiber 5, carbs 18.2, protein 12

Tilapia and Red Onion Mix

Preparation time: 10 minutes
Cooking time: 15 minutes
Servings: 4

Ingredients:
- 4 tilapia fillets, boneless
- 2 tablespoons olive oil
- 1 tablespoon lemon juice
- 2 teaspoons lemon zest, grated
- 2 red onions, roughly chopped
- 3 tablespoons chives, chopped

Directions:
1. Heat up a pan with the oil over medium heat, add the onions, lemon zest and lemon juice, toss and sauté for 5 minutes.
2. Add the fish and the chives, cook for 5 minutes on each side, divide between plates and serve.

Nutrition: calories 254, fat 18.2, fiber 5.4, carbs 11.7, protein 4.5

Trout Salad

Preparation time: 6 minutes
Cooking time: 0 minutes
Servings: 4

Ingredients:
- 4 ounces smoked trout, skinless, boneless and cubed
- 1 tablespoon lime juice
- 1/3 cup non-fat yogurt
- 2 avocados, peeled, pitted and cubed
- 3 tablespoons chives, chopped
- Black pepper to the taste
- 1 tablespoon olive oil

Directions:
1. In a bowl, combine the trout with the avocados and the other ingredients, toss, and serve.

Nutrition: calories 244, fat 9.45, fiber 5.6, carbs 8.5, protein 15

Balsamic Trout

Preparation time: 5 minutes
Cooking time: 15 minutes
Servings: 4

Ingredients:
- 3 tablespoons balsamic vinegar
- 2 tablespoons olive oil
- 4 trout fillets, boneless
- 3 tablespoons parsley, finely chopped
- 2 garlic cloves, minced

Directions:
1. Heat up a pan with the oil over medium heat, add the trout and cook for 6 minutes on each side.
2. Add the rest of the ingredients, cook for 3 minutes more, divide between plates and serve with a side salad.

Nutrition: calories 314, fat 14.3, fiber 8.2, carbs 14.8, protein 11.2

Parsley Salmon

Preparation time: 5 minutes
Cooking time: 12 minutes
Servings: 4

Ingredients:
- 2 spring onions, chopped
- 2 teaspoons lime juice
- 1 tablespoon chives, minced
- 1 tablespoon olive oil
- 4 salmon fillets, boneless
- Black pepper to the taste
- 2 tablespoons parsley, chopped

Directions:
1. Heat up a pan with the oil over medium heat, add the spring onions, stir and sauté for 2 minutes.
2. Add the salmon and the other ingredients, cook for 5 minutes on each side, divide between plates and serve.

Nutrition: calories 290, fat 14.4, fiber 5.6, carbs 15.6, protein 9.5

Trout and Veggie Salad

Preparation time: 5 minutes
Cooking time: 0 minutes
Servings: 4

Ingredients:
- 2 tablespoons olive oil
- ½ cup kalamata olives, pitted and minced
- Black pepper to the taste
- 1 pound smoked trout, boneless, skinless and cubed
- ½ teaspoon lemon zest, grated
- 1 tablespoon lemon juice
- 1 cup cherry tomatoes, halved
- ½ red onion, sliced
- 2 cups baby arugula

Directions:
1. In a bowl, combine smoked trout with the olives, black pepper and the other ingredients, toss and serve.

Nutrition: calories 282, fat 13.4, fiber 5.3, carbs 11.6, protein 5.6

Saffron Salmon

Preparation time: 10 minutes
Cooking time: 12 minutes
Servings: 4

Ingredients:
- Black pepper to the taste
- ½ teaspoon sweet paprika
- 4 salmon fillets, boneless
- 3 tablespoons olive oil
- 1 yellow onion, chopped
- 2 garlic cloves, minced
- ¼ teaspoon saffron powder

Directions:
1. Heat up a pan with the oil over medium-high heat, add the onion and the garlic, toss and sauté for 2 minutes.
2. Add the salmon and the other ingredients, cook for 5 minutes on each side, divide between plates and serve.

Nutrition: calories 339, fat 21.6, fiber 0.7, carbs 3.2, protein 35

Shrimp and Watermelon Salad

Preparation time: 10 minutes
Cooking time: 0 minutes
Servings: 4

Ingredients:
- ¼ cup basil, chopped
- 2 cups watermelon, peeled and cubed
- 2 tablespoons balsamic vinegar
- 2 tablespoons olive oil
- 1 pound shrimp, peeled, deveined and cooked
- Black pepper to the taste
- 1 tablespoon parsley, chopped

Directions:
1. In a bowl, combine the shrimp with the watermelon and the other ingredients, toss and serve.

Nutrition: calories 220, fat 9, fiber 0.4, carbs 7.6, protein 26.4

Oregano Shrimp and Quinoa Salad

Preparation time: 5 minutes
Cooking time: 8 minutes
Servings: 4

Ingredients:
- 1 pound shrimp, peeled and deveined
- 1 cup quinoa, cooked
- Black pepper to the taste
- 1 tablespoon olive oil
- 1 tablespoon oregano, chopped
- 1 red onion, chopped
- Juice of 1 lemon

Directions:
1. Heat up a pan with the oil over medium-high heat, add the onion, stir and sauté for 2 minutes.
2. Add the shrimp, toss and cook for 5 minutes.
3. Add the rest of the ingredients, toss, divide everything into bowls and serve.

Nutrition: calories 336, fat 8.2, fiber 4.1, carbs 32.3, protein 32.3

Crab Salad

Preparation time: 10 minutes
Cooking time: 0 minutes
Servings: 4

Ingredients:
- 1 tablespoon olive oil
- 2 cups crab meat
- Black pepper to the taste
- 1 cup cherry tomatoes, halved
- 1 shallot, chopped
- 1 tablespoon lemon juice
- 1/3 cup cilantro, chopped

Directions:
1. In a bowl, combine the crab with the tomatoes and the other ingredients, toss and serve.

Nutrition: calories 54, fat 3.9, fiber 0.6, carbs 2.6, protein 2.3

Balsamic Scallops

Preparation time: 4 minutes
Cooking time: 6 minutes
Servings: 4

Ingredients:
- 12 ounces sea scallops
- 2 tablespoons olive oil
- 2 garlic cloves, minced
- 1 tablespoon balsamic vinegar
- 1 cup scallions, sliced
- 2 tablespoons cilantro, chopped

Directions:
1. Heat up a pan with the oil over medium heat, add the scallions and the garlic and sauté for 2 minutes.
2. Add the scallops and the other ingredients, cook them for 2 minutes on each side, divide between plates and serve.

Nutrition: calories 146, fat 7.7, fiber 0.7, carbs 4.4, protein 14.8

Creamy Flounder Mix

Preparation time: 10 minutes
Cooking time: 20 minutes
Servings: 4

Ingredients:
- 2 tablespoon olive oil
- 1 red onion, chopped
- Black pepper to the taste
- ½ cup low-sodium veggie stock
- 4 flounder fillets, boneless
- ½ cup coconut cream
- 1 tablespoon dill, chopped

Directions:
1. Heat up a pan with the oil over medium heat, add the onion, stir and sauté for 5 minutes.
2. Add the fish and cook it for 4 minutes on each side.
3. Add the rest of the ingredients, cook for 7 minutes more, divide between plates and serve.

Nutrition: calories 232, fat 12.3, fiber 4, carbs 8.7, protein 12

Spicy Salmon and Mango Mix

Preparation time: 5 minutes
Cooking time: 0 minutes
Servings: 4

Ingredients:
- 1 pound smoked salmon, boneless, skinless and flaked
- Black pepper to the taste
- 1 red onion, chopped
- 1 mango, peeled, seedless and chopped
- 2 jalapeno peppers, chopped
- ¼ cup parsley, chopped
- 3 tablespoons lime juice
- 1 tablespoon olive oil

Directions:
2. In a bowl, mix the salmon with the black pepper and the other ingredients, toss and serve.

Nutrition: calories 323, fat 14.2, fiber 4, carbs 8.5, protein 20.4

Dill Shrimp Mix

Preparation time: 5 minutes
Cooking time: 0 minutes
Servings: 4

Ingredients:
- 2 teaspoons lemon juice
- 1 tablespoon olive oil
- 1 tablespoon dill, chopped
- 1 pound shrimp, cooked, peeled and deveined
- Black pepper to the taste
- 1 cup radishes, cubed

Directions:
1. In a bowl, combine the shrimp with the lemon juice and the other ingredients, toss and serve.

Nutrition: calories 292, fat 13, fiber 4.4, carbs 8, protein 16.4

Salmon Pate

Preparation time: 4 minutes
Cooking time: 0 minutes
Servings: 6

Ingredients:
- 6 ounces smoked salmon, boneless, skinless and shredded
- 2 tablespoons non-fat yogurt
- 3 teaspoons lemon juice
- 2 spring onions, chopped
- 8 ounces low-fat cream cheese
- ¼ cup cilantro, chopped

Directions:
1. In a bowl, mix the salmon with the yogurt and the other ingredients, whisk and serve cold.

Nutrition: calories 272, fat 15.2, fiber 4.3, carbs 16.8, protein 9.9

Shrimp with Artichokes

Preparation time: 4 minutes
Cooking time: 8 minutes
Servings: 4

Ingredients:
- 2 green onions, chopped
- 1 cup canned artichokes, no-salt-added, drained and quartered
- 2 tablespoons cilantro, chopped
- 1 pound shrimp, peeled and deveined
- 1 cup cherry tomatoes, cubed
- 1 tablespoon olive oil
- 1 tablespoon balsamic vinegar
- A pinch of salt and black pepper

Directions:
1. Heat up a pan with the oil over medium heat, add the onions and the artichokes, toss and cook for 2 minutes.
2. Add the shrimp, toss and cook over medium heat for 6 minutes.
3. Divide everything into bowls and serve.

Nutrition: calories 260, fat 8.23, fiber 3.8, carbs 14.3, protein 12.4

Shrimp with Lemon Sauce

Preparation time: 5 minutes
Cooking time: 8 minutes
Servings: 4

Ingredients:
- 1 pound shrimp, peeled and deveined
- 2 tablespoons olive oil
- Zest of 1 lemon, grated
- Juice of ½ lemon
- 1 tablespoon chives, chopped

Directions:
1. Heat up a pan with the oil over medium-high heat, add the lemon zest, lemon juice and the cilantro, toss and cook for 2 minutes.
2. Add the shrimp, cook everything for 6 minutes more, divide between plates and serve.

Nutrition: calories 195, fat 8.9, fiber 0, carbs 1.8, protein 25.9

Tuna and Orange Mix

Preparation time: 5 minutes
Cooking time: 12 minutes
Servings: 4

Ingredients:
- 4 tuna fillets, boneless
- Black pepper to the taste
- 2 tablespoons olive oil
- 2 shallots, chopped
- 3 tablespoons orange juice
- 1 orange, peeled and cut into segments
- 1 tablespoon oregano, chopped

Directions:
1. Heat up a pan with the oil over medium-high heat, add the shallots, stir and sauté for 2 minutes.
2. Add the tuna and the other ingredients, cook everything for 10 minutes more, divide between plates and serve.

Nutrition: calories 457, fat 38.2, fiber 1.6, carbs 8.2, protein 21.8

Salmon Curry

Preparation time: 10 minutes
Cooking time: 20 minutes
Servings: 4

Ingredients:
- 1 pound salmon fillet, boneless and cubed
- 3 tablespoons red curry paste
- 1 red onion, chopped
- 1 teaspoon sweet paprika
- 1 cup coconut cream
- 1 tablespoon olive oil
- Black pepper to the taste
- ½ cup low-sodium chicken stock
- 3 tablespoons basil, chopped

Directions:
1. Heat up a pan with the oil over medium-high heat, add the onion, paprika and the curry paste, toss and cook for 5 minutes.
2. Add the salmon and the other ingredients, toss gently, cook over medium heat for 15 minutes, divide into bowls and serve.

Nutrition: calories 377, fat 28.3, fiber 2.1, carbs 8.5, protein 23.9

Salmon and Carrots Mix

Preparation time: 10 minutes
Cooking time: 15 minutes
Servings: 4

Ingredients:
- 4 salmon fillets, boneless
- 1 red onion, chopped
- 2 carrots, sliced
- 2 tablespoons olive oil
- 2 tablespoons balsamic vinegar
- Black pepper to the taste
- 2 tablespoons chives, chopped
- ¼ cup low-sodium veggie stock

Directions:
1. Heat up a pan with the oil over medium heat, add the onion and the carrots, toss and sauté for 5 minutes.
2. Add the salmon and the other ingredients, cook everything for 10 minutes more, divide between plates and serve.

Nutrition: calories 322, fat 18, fiber 1.4, carbs 6, protein 35.2

Shrimp and Pine Nuts Mix

Preparation time: 10 minutes
Cooking time: 10 minutes
Servings: 4

Ingredients:
- 1 pound shrimp, peeled and deveined
- 2 tablespoons pine nuts
- 1 tablespoon lime juice
- 2 tablespoons olive oil
- 3 garlic cloves, minced
- Black pepper to the taste
- 1 tablespoon thyme, chopped
- 2 tablespoons chives, finely chopped

Directions:
1. Heat up a pan with the oil over medium-high heat, add the garlic, thyme, pine nuts and lime juice, toss and cook for 3 minutes.
2. Add the shrimp, black pepper and the chives, toss, cook for 7 minutes more, divide between plates and serve.

Nutrition: calories 290, fat 13, fiber 4.5, carbs 13.9, protein 10

Chili Cod and Green Beans

Preparation time: 10 minutes
Cooking time: 14 minutes
Servings: 4

Ingredients:
- 4 cod fillets, boneless
- ½ pound green beans, trimmed and halved
- 1 tablespoon lime juice
- 1 tablespoon lime zest, grated
- 1 yellow onion, chopped
- 2 tablespoons olive oil
- 1 teaspoon cumin, ground
- 1 teaspoon chili powder
- ½ cup low-sodium veggie stock
- A pinch of salt and black pepper

Directions:
1. Heat up a pan with the oil over medium-high heat, add the onion, toss and cook for 2 minutes.
2. Add the fish and cook it for 3 minutes on each side.
3. Add the green beans and the rest of the ingredients, toss gently, cook for 7 minutes more, divide between plates and serve.

Nutrition: calories 220, fat 13, carbs 14.3, fiber 2.3, protein 12

Garlic Scallops

Preparation time: 5 minutes
Cooking time: 8 minutes
Servings: 4

Ingredients:
- 12 scallops
- 1 red onion, sliced
- 2 tablespoons olive oil
- ½ teaspoon garlic, minced
- 2 tablespoons lemon juice
- Black pepper to the taste
- 1 teaspoon balsamic vinegar

Directions:
1. Heat up a pan with the oil over medium heat, add the onion and the garlic and sauté for 2 minutes.
2. Add the scallops and the other ingredients, cook over medium heat for 6 minutes more, divide between plates and serve hot.

Nutrition: calories 259, fat 8, fiber 3, carbs 5.7, protein 7

Creamy Sea Bass Mix

Preparation time: 10 minutes
Cooking time: 14 minutes
Servings: 4

Ingredients:
- 4 sea bass fillets, boneless
- 1 cup coconut cream
- 1 yellow onion, chopped
- 1 tablespoon lime juice
- 2 tablespoons avocado oil
- 1 tablespoon parsley, chopped
- A pinch of black pepper

Directions:
1. Heat up a pan with the oil over medium heat, add the onion, toss and sauté for 2 minutes.
2. Add the fish and cook it for 4 minutes on each side.
3. Add the rest of the ingredients, cook everything for 4 minutes more, divide between plates and serve.

Nutrition: calories 283, fat 12.3, fiber 5, carbs 12.5, protein 8

Sea Bass and Mushrooms Mix

Preparation time: 10 minutes
Cooking time: 13 minutes
Servings: 4

Ingredients:
- 4 sea bass fillets, boneless
- 2 tablespoons olive oil
- Black pepper to the taste
- ½ cup white mushrooms, sliced
- 1 red onion, chopped
- 2 tablespoons balsamic vinegar
- 3 tablespoons cilantro, chopped

Directions:
1. Heat up a pan with the oil over medium-high heat, add the onion and the mushrooms, stir and cook for 5 minutes.
2. Add the fish and the other ingredients, cook for 4 minutes on each side, divide everything between plates and serve.

Nutrition: calories 280, fat 12.3, fiber 8, carbs 13.6, protein 14.3

Salmon Chowder

Preparation time: 5 minutes
Cooking time: 20 minutes
Servings: 4

Ingredients:

- 1 pound salmon fillets, boneless, skinless and cubed
- 1 cup yellow onion, chopped
- 2 tablespoons olive oil
- Black pepper to the taste
- 2 cups low-sodium veggie stock
- 1 and ½ cups tomatoes, chopped
- 1 tablespoon basil, chopped

Directions:

1. Heat up a pot with the oil over medium heat, add the onion, stir and sauté for 5 minutes.
2. Add the salmon and the other ingredients, bring to a simmer and cook over medium heat for 15 minutes.
3. Divide the chowder into bowls and serve.

Nutrition: calories 250, fat 12.2, fiber 5, carbs 8.5, protein 7

Nutmeg Shrimp

Preparation time: 3 minutes
Cooking time: 6 minutes
Servings: 4

Ingredients:
- 1 pound shrimp, peeled and deveined
- 2 tablespoons olive oil
- 1 tablespoon lemon juice
- 1 tablespoon nutmeg, ground
- Black pepper to the taste
- 1 tablespoon cilantro, chopped

Directions:
1. Heat up a pan with the oil over medium heat, add the shrimp, lemon juice and the other ingredients, toss, cook for 6 minutes, divide into bowls and serve.

Nutrition: calories 205, fat 9.6, fiber 0.4, carbs 2.7, protein 26

Shrimp and Berries Mix

Preparation time: 4 minutes
Cooking time: 6 minutes
Servings: 4

Ingredients:
- 1 pound shrimp, peeled and deveined
- ½ cup tomatoes, cubed
- 2 tablespoons olive oil
- 1 tablespoon balsamic vinegar
- ½ cup strawberries, chopped
- Black pepper to the taste

Directions:
1. Heat up a pan with the oil over medium heat, add the shrimp, toss and cook for 3 minutes.
2. Add the rest of the ingredients, toss, cook for 3-4 minutes more, divide into bowls and serve.

Nutrition: calories 205, fat 9, fiber 0.6, carbs 4, protein 26.2

Baked Lemony Trout

Preparation time: 10 minutes
Cooking time: 30 minutes
Servings: 4

Ingredients:
- 4 trout
- 1 tablespoon lemon zest, grated
- 2 tablespoons olive oil
- 2 tablespoons lemon juice
- A pinch of black pepper
- 2 tablespoons cilantro, chopped

Directions:
1. In a baking dish, combine the fish with the lemon zest and the other ingredients and rub.
2. Bake at 370 degrees F for 30 minutes, divide between plates and serve.

Nutrition: calories 264, fat 12.3, fiber 5, carbs 7, protein 11

Chives Scallops

Preparation time: 3 minutes
Cooking time: 4 minutes
Servings: 4

Ingredients:
- 12 scallops
- 2 tablespoons olive oil
- Black pepper to the taste
- 2 tablespoons chives, chopped
- 1 tablespoon sweet paprika

Directions:
1. Heat up a pan with the oil over medium heat, add the scallops, paprika and the other ingredients, and cook for 2 minutes on each side.
2. Divide between plates and serve with a side salad.

Nutrition: calories 215, fat 6, fiber 5, carbs 4.5, protein 11

Tuna Meatballs

Preparation time: 10 minutes
Cooking time: 30 minutes
Servings: 4

Ingredients:
- 2 tablespoons olive oil
- 1 pound tuna, skinless, boneless and minced
- 1 yellow onion, chopped
- ¼ cup chives, chopped
- 1 egg, whisked
- 1 tablespoon coconut flour
- A pinch of salt and black pepper

Directions:
1. In a bowl, mix the tuna with the onion and the other ingredients except the oil, stir well and shape medium meatballs out of this mix.
2. Arrange the meatballs on a baking sheet, grease them with the oil, introduce in the oven at 350 degrees F, cook for 30 minutes, divide between plates and serve.

Nutrition: calories 291, fat 14.3, fiber 5, carbs 12.4, protein 11

Salmon Pan

Preparation time: 10 minutes
Cooking time: 12 minutes
Servings: 4

Ingredients:
- 4 salmon fillets, boneless and roughly cubed
- 2 tablespoons olive oil
- 1 red bell pepper, cut into strips
- 1 zucchini, roughly cubed
- 1 eggplant, roughly cubed
- 1 tablespoon lemon juice
- 1 tablespoon dill, chopped
- ¼ cup low-sodium veggie stock
- 1 teaspoon garlic powder
- A pinch of black pepper

Directions:
1. Heat up a pan with oil over medium-high heat, add the bell pepper, zucchini and the eggplant, toss and sauté for 3 minutes.
2. Add the salmon and the other ingredients, toss gently, cook everything for 9 minutes more, divide between plates and serve.

Nutrition: calories 348, fat 18.4, fiber 5.3, carbs 11.9, protein 36.9

Mustard Cod Mix

Preparation time: 10 minutes
Cooking time: 25 minutes
Servings: 4

Ingredients:
- 4 cod fillets, skinless and boneless
- A pinch of black pepper
- 1 teaspoon ginger, grated
- 1 tablespoon mustard
- 2 tablespoons olive oil
- 1 teaspoon thyme, dried
- ¼ teaspoon cumin, ground
- 1 teaspoon turmeric powder
- ¼ cup cilantro, chopped
- 1 cup low-sodium veggie stock
- 3 garlic cloves, minced

Directions:
1. In a roasting pan, combine the cod with the black pepper, ginger and the other ingredients, toss gently and bake at 380 degrees F for 25 minutes.
2. Divide the mix between plates and serve.

Nutrition: calories 176, fat 9, fiber 1, carbs 3.7, protein 21.2

Shrimp and Asparagus Mix

Preparation time: 10 minutes
Cooking time: 14 minutes
Servings: 4

Ingredients:
- 1 asparagus bunch, halved
- 1 pound shrimp, peeled and deveined
- Black pepper to the taste
- 2 tablespoons olive oil
- 1 red onion, chopped
- 2 garlic cloves, minced
- 1 cup coconut cream

Directions:
1. Heat up a pan with the oil over medium heat, add the onion, garlic and the asparagus, toss and cook for 4 minutes.
2. Add the shrimp and the other ingredients, toss, simmer over medium heat for 10 minutes, divide everything into bowls and serve.

Nutrition: calories 225, fat 6, fiber 3.4, carbs 8.6, protein 8

Cod and Peas

Preparation time: 10 minutes
Cooking time: 20 minutes
Servings: 4

Ingredients:
- 1 yellow onion, chopped
- 2 tablespoons olive oil
- ½ cup low-sodium chicken stock
- 4 cod fillets, boneless, skinless
- Black pepper to the taste
- 1 cup snow peas

Directions:
1. Heat up a pot with the oil over medium heat, add the onion, stir and sauté fro 4 minutes.
2. Add the fish and cook it for 3 minutes on each side.
3. Add the snow peas and the other ingredients, cook everything for 10 minutes more, divide between plates and serve.

Nutrition: calories 240, fat 8.4, fiber 2.7, carbs 7.6, protein 14

Shrimp and Mussels Bowls

Preparation time: 5 minutes
Cooking time: 12 minutes
Servings: 4

Ingredients:
- 1 pound mussels, scrubbed
- ½ cup low-sodium chicken stock
- 1 pound shrimp, peeled and deveined
- 2 shallots, minced
- 1 cup cherry tomatoes, cubed
- 2 garlic cloves, minced
- 1 tablespoon olive oil
- Juice of 1 lemon

Directions:
1. Heat up a pan with the oil over medium heat, add the shallots and the garlic and sauté for 2 minutes.
2. Add the shrimp, mussels and the other ingredients, cook everything over medium heat for 10 minutes, divide into bowls and serve.

Nutrition: calories 240, fat 4.9, fiber 2.4, carbs 11.6, protein 8

Dash Diet Dessert Recipes

Mint Cream

Preparation time: 2 hours and 4 minutes

Cooking time: 0 minutes
Servings: 4

Ingredients:
- 4 cups non-fat yogurt
- 1 cup coconut cream
- 3 tablespoons stevia
- 2 teaspoons lime zest, grated
- 1 tablespoon mint, chopped

Directions:
1. In a blender, combine the cream with the yogurt and the other ingredients, pulse well, divide into cups and keep in the fridge for 2 hours before serving.

Nutrition: calories 512, fat 14.3, fiber 1.5, carbs 83.6, protein 12.1

Raspberries Pudding

Preparation time: 10 minutes
Cooking time: 24 minutes
Servings: 4

Ingredients:
- 1 cup raspberries
- 2 teaspoons coconut sugar
- 3 eggs, whisked
- 1 tablespoon avocado oil
- ½ cup almond milk
- ½ cup coconut flour
- ¼ cup non-fat yogurt

Directions:
1. In a bowl, combine the raspberries with the sugar and the other ingredients except the cooking spray and whisk well.
2. Grease a pudding pan with the cooking spray, add the raspberries mix, spread, bake in the oven at 400 degrees F for 24 minutes, divide between dessert plates and serve.

Nutrition: calories 215, fat 11.3, fiber 3.4, carbs 21.3, protein 6.7

Almond Bars

Preparation time: 10 minutes
Cooking time: 30 minutes
Servings: 4

Ingredients:
- 1 cup almonds, crushed
- 2 eggs, whisked
- ½ cup almond milk
- 1 teaspoon vanilla extract
- 2/3 cup coconut sugar
- 2 cups whole flour
- 1 teaspoon baking powder
- Cooking spray

Directions:
1. In a bowl, combine the almonds with the eggs and the other ingredients except the cooking spray and stir well.
2. Pour this into a square pan greased with cooking spray, spread well, bake in the oven for 30 minutes, cool down, cut into bars and serve.

Nutrition: calories 463, fat 22.5, fiber 11, carbs 54.4, protein 16.9

Baked Peaches Mix

Preparation time: 10 minutes
Cooking time: 30 minutes
Servings: 4

Ingredients:
- 4 peaches, stones removed and halved
- 1 tablespoon coconut sugar
- 1 teaspoon vanilla extract
- ¼ teaspoon cinnamon powder
- 1 tablespoon avocado oil

Directions:
1. In a baking pan, combine the peaches with the sugar and the other ingredients, bake at 375 degrees F for 30 minutes, cool down and serve.

Nutrition: calories 91, fat 0.8, fiber 2.5, carb 19.2, protein 1.7

Walnuts Cake

Preparation time: 10 minutes
Cooking time: 25 minutes
Servings: 8

Ingredients:
- 3 cups almond flour
- 1 cup coconut sugar
- 1 tablespoon vanilla extract
- ½ cup walnuts, chopped
- 2 teaspoons baking soda
- 2 cups coconut milk
- ½ cup coconut oil, melted

Directions:
1. In a bowl, combine the almond flour with the sugar and the other ingredients, whisk well, pour into a cake pan, spread, introduce in the oven at 370 degrees F, bake for 25 minutes.
2. Leave the cake to cool down, slice and serve.

Nutrition: calories 445, fat 10, fiber 6.5, carbs 31.4, protein 23.5

Apple Cake

Preparation time: 10 minutes
Cooking time: 30 minutes
Servings: 4

Ingredients:
- 2 cups almond flour
- 1 teaspoon baking soda
- 1 teaspoon baking powder
- ½ teaspoon cinnamon powder
- 2 tablespoons coconut sugar
- 1 cup almond milk
- 2 green apples, cored, peeled and chopped
- Cooking spray

Directions:
1. In a bowl, combine the flour with the baking soda, the apples and the other ingredients except the cooking spray, and whisk well.
2. Pour this into a cake pan greased with the cooking spray, spread well, introduce in the oven and bake at 360 degrees F for 30 minutes.
3. Cool the cake down, slice and serve.

Nutrition: calories 332, fat 22.4, fiber 9l.6, carbs 22.2, protein 12.3

Cinnamon Cream

Preparation time: 2 hours
Cooking time: 10 minutes
Servings: 4

Ingredients:
- 1 cup non-fat almond milk
- 1 cup coconut cream
- 2 cups coconut sugar
- 2 tablespoons cinnamon powder
- 1 teaspoon vanilla extract

Directions:
1. Heat up a pan with the almond milk over medium heat, add the rest of the ingredients, whisk, and cook for 10 minutes more.
2. Divide the mix into bowls, cool down and keep in the fridge for 2 hours before serving.

Nutrition: calories 254, fat 7.5, fiber 5, carbs 16.4, protein 9.5

Creamy Strawberries Mix

Preparation time: 10 minutes
Cooking time: 0 minutes
Servings: 4

Ingredients:
- 1 teaspoon vanilla extract
- 2 cups strawberries, chopped
- 1 teaspoon coconut sugar
- 8 ounces non-fat yogurt

Directions:
1. In a bowl, combine the strawberries with the vanilla and the other ingredients, toss and serve cold.

Nutrition: calories 343, fat 13.4, fiber 6, carb 15.43, protein 5.5

Vanilla Pecan Brownies

Preparation time: 10 minutes
Cooking time: 25 minutes
Servings: 8

Ingredients:
- 1 cup pecans, chopped
- 3 tablespoons coconut sugar
- 2 tablespoons cocoa powder
- 3 eggs, whisked
- ¼ cup coconut oil, melted
- ½ teaspoon baking powder
- 2 teaspoons vanilla extract
- Cooking spray

Directions:
1. In your food processor, combine the pecans with the coconut sugar and the other ingredients except the cooking spray and pulse well.
2. Grease a square pan with cooking spray, add the brownies mix, spread, introduce in the oven, bake at 350 degrees F for 25 minutes, leave aside to cool down, slice and serve.

Nutrition: calories 370, fat 14.3, fiber 3, carbs 14.4, protein 5.6

Strawberries Cake

Preparation time: 10 minutes
Cooking time: 25 minutes
Servings: 6

Ingredients:
- 2 cups whole wheat flour
- 1 cup strawberries, chopped
- ½ teaspoon baking soda
- ½ cup coconut sugar
- ¾ cup coconut milk
- ¼ cup coconut oil, melted
- 2 eggs, whisked
- 1 teaspoon vanilla extract
- Cooking spray

Directions:
1. In a bowl, combine the flour with the strawberries and the other ingredients except the coking spray and whisk well.
2. Grease a cake pan with cooking spray, pour the cake mix, spread, bake in the oven at 350 degrees F for 25 minutes, cool down, slice and serve.

Nutrition: calories 465, fat 22.1, fiber 4, carbs 18.3, protein 13.4

Cocoa Pudding

Preparation time: 10 minutes
Cooking time: 10 minutes
Servings: 4

Ingredients:
- 2 tablespoons coconut sugar
- 3 tablespoons coconut flour
- 2 tablespoons cocoa powder
- 2 cups almond milk
- 2 eggs, whisked
- ½ teaspoon vanilla extract

Directions:
1. Put the milk in a pan, add the cocoa and the other ingredients, whisk, simmer over medium heat for 10 minutes, pour into small cups and serve cold.

Nutrition: calories 385, fat 31.7, fiber 5.7, carbs 21.6, protein 7.3

Nutmeg Vanilla Cream

Preparation time: 10 minutes
Cooking time: 0 minutes
Servings: 6

Ingredients:
- 3 cups non-fat milk
- 1 teaspoon nutmeg, ground
- 2 teaspoons vanilla extract
- 4 teaspoons coconut sugar
- 1 cup walnuts, chopped

Directions:
1. In a bowl, combine milk with the nutmeg and the other ingredients, whisk well, divide into small cups and serve cold.

Nutrition: calories 243, fat 12.4, fiber 1.5, carbs 21.1, protein 9.7

Avocado Cream

Preparation time: 1 hour and 10 minutes

Cooking time: 0 minutes
Servings: 4

Ingredients:
- 2 cups coconut cream
- 2 avocados, peeled, pitted and mashed
- 2 tablespoons coconut sugar
- 1 teaspoon vanilla extract

Directions:
1. In a blender, combine the cream with the avocados and the other ingredients, pulse well, divide into cups and keep in the fridge for 1 hour before serving.

Nutrition: calories 532, fat 48.2, fiber 9.4, carbs 24.9, protein 5.2

Raspberries Cream

Preparation time: 10 minutes
Cooking time: 25 minutes
Servings: 4

Ingredients:
- 2 tablespoons almond flour
- 1 cup coconut cream
- 3 cups raspberries
- 1 cup coconut sugar
- 8 ounces low-fat cream cheese

Directions:
1. In a bowl, the flour with the cream and the other ingredients, whisk, transfer to a round pan, cook at 360 degrees F for 25 minutes, divide into bowls and serve.

Nutrition: calories 429, fat 36.3, fiber 7.7, carbs 21.3, protein 7.8

Watermelon Salad

Preparation time: 4 minutes
Cooking time: 0 minutes
Servings: 4

Ingredients:
- 1 cup watermelon, peeled and cubed
- 2 apples, cored and cubed
- 1 tablespoon coconut cream
- 2 bananas, cut into chunks

Directions:
1. In a bowl, combine the watermelon with the apples and the other ingredients, toss and serve.

Nutrition: calories 131, fat 1.3, fiber 4.5, carbs 31.9, protein 1.3

Coconut Pears Mix

Preparation time: 10 minutes
Cooking time: 10 minutes
Servings: 4

Ingredients:
- 2 teaspoons lime juice
- ½ cup coconut cream
- ½ cup coconut, shredded
- 4 pears, cored and cubed
- 4 tablespoons coconut sugar

Directions:
1. In a pan, combine the pears with the lime juice and the other ingredients, stir, bring to a simmer over medium heat and cook for 10 minutes.
2. Divide into bowls and serve cold.

Nutrition: calories 320, fat 7.8, fiber 3, carbs 6.4, protein 4.7

Apples Compote

Preparation time: 10 minutes
Cooking time: 15 minutes
Servings: 4

Ingredients:
- 5 tablespoons coconut sugar
- 2 cups orange juice
- 4 apples, cored and cubed

Directions:
1. In a pot, combine apples with the sugar and the orange juice, toss, bring to a boil over medium heat, cook for 15 minutes, divide into bowls and serve cold.

Nutrition: calories 220, fat 5.2, fiber 3, carbs 5.6, protein 5.6

Apricots Stew

Preparation time: 10 minutes
Cooking time: 15 minutes
Servings: 4

Ingredients:
- 2 cups apricots, halved
- 2 cups water
- 2 tablespoons coconut sugar
- 2 tablespoons lemon juice

Directions:
1. In a pot, combine the apricots with the water and the other ingredients, toss, cook over medium heat for 15 minutes, divide into bowls and serve.

Nutrition: calories 260, fat 6.2, fiber 4.2, carbs 5.6, protein 6

Lemon Cantaloupe Mix

Preparation time: 10 minutes
Cooking time: 10 minutes
Servings: 4

Ingredients:
- 2 cups cantaloupe, peeled and roughly cubed
- 4 tablespoons coconut sugar
- 2 teaspoons vanilla extract
- 2 teaspoons lemon juice

Directions:
1. In a small pan, combine the cantaloupe with the sugar and the other ingredients, toss, heat up over medium heat, cook for about 10 minutes, divide into bowls and serve cold.

Nutrition: calories 140, fat 4, fiber 3.4, carbs 6.7, protein 5

Creamy Rhubarb Cream

Preparation time: 10 minutes
Cooking time: 14 minutes
Servings: 4

Ingredients:
- 1/3 cup low-fat cream cheese
- ½ cup coconut cream
- 2 pound rhubarb, roughly chopped
- 3 tablespoons coconut sugar

Directions:
1. In a blender, combine the cream cheese with the cream and the other ingredients and pulse well.
2. Divide into small cups, introduce in the oven and bake at 350 degrees F for 14 minutes.
3. Serve cold.

Nutrition: calories 360, fat 14.3, fiber 4.4, carbs 5.8, protein 5.2

Pineapple Bowls

Preparation time: 10 minutes
Cooking time: 0 minutes
Servings: 4

Ingredients:

- 3 cups pineapple, peeled and cubed
- 1 teaspoon chia seeds
- 1 cup coconut cream
- 1 teaspoon vanilla extract
- 1 tablespoon mint, chopped

Directions:

1. In a bowl, combine the pineapple with the cream and the other ingredients, toss, divide into smaller bowls and keep in the fridge for 10 minutes before serving.

Nutrition: calories 238, fat 16.6, fiber 5.6, carbs 22.8, protein 3.3

Blueberry Stew

Preparation time: 10 minutes
Cooking time: 10 minutes
Servings: 4

Ingredients:
- 2 tablespoons lemon juice
- 1 cup water
- 3 tablespoons coconut sugar
- 12 ounces blueberries

Directions:
1. In a pan, combine the blueberries with the sugar and the other ingredients, bring to a gentle simmer and cook over medium heat for 10 minutes.
2. Divide into bowls and serve.

Nutrition: calories 122, fat 0.4, fiber 2.1, carbs 26.7, protein 1.5

Lime Pudding

Preparation time: 10 minutes
Cooking time: 15 minutes
Servings: 4

Ingredients:
- 2 cups coconut cream
- Juice of 1 lime
- Zest of 1 lime, grated
- 3 tablespoons coconut oil, melted
- 1 egg, whisked
- 1 teaspoon baking powder

Directions:
1. In a bowl, combine the cream with the lime juice and the other ingredients and whisk well.
2. Divide into small ramekins, introduce in the oven and bake at 360 degrees F for 15 minutes.
3. Serve the pudding cold.

Nutrition: calories 385, fat 39.9, fiber 2.7, carbs 8.2, protein 4.2

Peach Cream

Preparation time: 10 minutes
Cooking time: 0 minutes
Servings: 4

Ingredients:
- 3 cups coconut cream
- 2 peaches, stones removed and chopped
- 1 teaspoon vanilla extract
- ½ cup almonds, chopped

Directions:
1. In a blender, combine the cream and the other ingredients, pulse well, divide into small bowls and serve cold.

Nutrition: calories 261, fat 13, fiber 5.6, carbs 7, protein 5.4

Cinnamon Plums Mix

Preparation time: 10 minutes
Cooking time: 15 minutes
Servings: 4

Ingredients:
- 1 pound plums, stones removed and halved
- 2 tablespoons coconut sugar
- ½ teaspoon cinnamon powder
- 1 cup water

Directions:
1. In a pan, combine the plums with the sugar and the other ingredients, bring to a simmer and cook over medium heat for 15 minutes.
2. Divide into bowls and serve cold.

Nutrition: calories 142, fat 4, fiber 2.4, carbs 14, protein 7

Chia and Vanilla Apples

Preparation time: 10 minutes
Cooking time: 10 minutes
Servings: 4

Ingredients:
- 2 cups apples, cored and cut into wedges
- 2 tablespoons chia seeds
- 1 teaspoon vanilla extract
- 2 cups naturally unsweetened apple juice

Directions:
1. In a small pot, combine the apples with the chia seeds and the other ingredients, toss, cook over medium heat for 10 minutes, divide into bowls and serve cold.

Nutrition: calories 172, fat 5.6, fiber 3.5, carbs 10, protein 4.4

Rice and Pears Pudding

Preparation time: 10 minutes
Cooking time: 25 minutes
Servings: 4

Ingredients:
- 6 cups water
- 1 cup coconut sugar
- 2 cups black rice
- 2 pears, cored and cubed
- 2 teaspoons cinnamon powder

Directions:
1. Put the water in a pan, heat it up over medium-high heat, add the rice, sugar and the other ingredients, stir, bring to a simmer, reduce heat to medium and cook for 25 minutes.
2. Divide into bowls and serve cold.

Nutrition: calories 290, fat 13.4, fiber 4, carbs 13.20, protein 6.7

Rhubarb Stew

Preparation time: 10 minutes
Cooking time: 15 minutes
Servings: 4

Ingredients:
- 2 cups rhubarb, roughly chopped
- 3 tablespoons coconut sugar
- 1 teaspoon almond extract
- 2 cups water

Directions:
1. In a pot, combine the rhubarb with the other ingredients, toss, bring to a boil over medium heat, cook for 15 minutes, divide into bowls and serve cold.

Nutrition: calories 142, fat 4.1, fiber 4.2, carbs 7, protein 4

Rhubarb Cream

Preparation time: 1 hour
Cooking time: 10 minutes
Servings: 4

Ingredients:
- 2 cups coconut cream
- 1 cup rhubarb, chopped
- 3 eggs, whisked
- 3 tablespoons coconut sugar
- 1 tablespoon lime juice

Directions:
1. In a small pan, combine the cream with the rhubarb and the other ingredients, whisk well, simmer over medium heat for 10 minutes, blend using an immersion blender, divide into bowls and keep in the fridge for 1 hour before serving.

Nutrition: calories 230, fat 8.4, fiber 2.4, carbs 7.8, protein 6

Blueberries Salad

Preparation time: 5 minutes
Cooking time: 0 minutes
Servings: 4

Ingredients:
- 2 cups blueberries
- 3 tablespoons mint, chopped
- 1 pear, cored and cubed
- 1 apple, core and cubed
- 1 tablespoon coconut sugar

Directions:
1. In a bowl, combine the blueberries with the mint and the other ingredients, toss and serve cold.

Nutrition: calories 150, fat 2.4, fiber 4, carbs 6.8, protein 6

Dates and Banana Cream

Preparation time: 5 minutes
Cooking time: 0 minutes
Servings: 4

Ingredients:
- 1 cup almond milk
- 1 banana, peeled and sliced
- 1 teaspoon vanilla extract
- ½ cup coconut cream
- dates, chopped

Directions:
1. In a blender, combine the dates with the banana and the other ingredients, pulse well, divide into small cups and serve cold.

Nutrition: calories 271, fat 21.6, fiber 3.8, carbs 21.2, protein 2.7

Plum Muffins

Preparation time: 10 minutes
Cooking time: 25 minutes
Servings: 12

Ingredients:
- 3 tablespoons coconut oil, melted
- ½ cup almond milk
- 4 eggs, whisked
- 1 teaspoon vanilla extract
- 1 cup almond flour
- 2 teaspoons cinnamon powder
- ½ teaspoon baking powder
- 1 cup plums, pitted and chopped

Directions:
1. In a bowl, combine the coconut oil with the almond milk and the other ingredients and whisk well.
2. Divide into a muffin pan, introduce in the oven at 350 degrees F and bake for 25 minutes.
3. Serve the muffins cold.

Nutrition: calories 270, fat 3.4, fiber 4.4, carbs 12, protein 5

Plums and Raisins Bowls

Preparation time: 10 minutes
Cooking time: 20 minutes
Servings: 4

Ingredients:
- ½ pound plums, pitted and halved
- 2 tablespoons coconut sugar
- 4 tablespoons raisins
- 1 teaspoon vanilla extract
- 1 cup coconut cream

Directions:
1. In a pan, combine the plums with the sugar and the other ingredients, bring to a simmer and cook over medium heat for 20 minutes.
2. Divide into bowls and serve.

Nutrition: calories 219, fat 14.4, fiber 1.8, carbs 21.1, protein 2.2

Sunflower Seed Bars

Preparation time: 10 minutes
Cooking time: 20 minutes
Servings: 6

Ingredients:
- 1 cup coconut flour
- ½ teaspoon baking soda
- 1 tablespoon flax seed
- 3 tablespoons almond milk
- 1 cup sunflower seeds
- 2 tablespoons coconut oil, melted
- 1 teaspoon vanilla extract

Directions:
1. In a bowl, mix the flour with the baking soda and the other ingredients, stir really well, spread on a baking sheet, press well, bake in the oven at 350 degrees F for 20 minutes, leave aside to cool down, cut into bars and serve.

Nutrition: calories 189, fat 12.6, fiber 9.2, carbs 15.7, protein 4.7

Blackberries and Cashews Bowls

Preparation time: 10 minutes
Cooking time: 0 minutes
Servings: 4
Ingredients:

- 1 cup cashews
- 2 cups blackberries
- ¾ cup coconut cream
- 1 teaspoon vanilla extract
- 1 tablespoon coconut sugar

Directions:

1. In a bowl, combine the cashews with the berries and the other ingredients, toss, divide into small bowls and serve.

Nutrition: calories 230, fat 4, fiber 3.4, carbs 12.3, protein 8

Orange and Mandarins Bowls

Preparation time: 4 minutes
Cooking time: 8 minutes
Servings: 4

Ingredients:
- 4 oranges, peeled and cut into segments
- 2 mandarins, peeled and cut into segments
- Juice of 1 lime
- 2 tablespoons coconut sugar
- 1 cup water

Directions:
1. In a pan, combine the oranges with the mandarins and the other ingredients, bring to a simmer and cook over medium heat for 8 minutes.
2. Divide into bowls and serve cold.

Nutrition: calories 170, fat 2.3, fiber 2.3, carbs 11, protein 3.4

Pumpkin Cream

Preparation time: 2 hours
Cooking time: 0 minutes
Servings: 4

Ingredients:
- 2 cups coconut cream
- 1 cup pumpkin puree
- 14 ounces coconut cream
- 3 tablespoons coconut sugar

Directions:
1. In a bowl, combine the cream with the pumpkin puree and the other ingredients, whisk well, divide into small bowls and keep in the fridge for 2 hours before serving.

Nutrition: calories 350, fat 12.3, fiber 3, carbs 11.7, protein 6

Figs and Rhubarb Mix

Preparation time: 6 minutes
Cooking time: 14 minutes
Servings: 4

Ingredients:
- 2 tablespoons coconut oil, melted
- 1 cup rhubarb, roughly chopped
- 12 figs, halved
- ¼ cup coconut sugar
- 1 cup water

Directions:
1. Heat up a pan with the oil over medium heat, add the figs and the rest of the ingredients, toss, cook for 14 minutes, divide into small cups and serve cold.

Nutrition: calories 213, fat 7.4, fiber 6.1, carbs 39, protein 2.2

Spiced Banana

Preparation time: 4 minutes
Cooking time: 15 minutes
Servings: 4

Ingredients:
- 4 bananas, peeled and halved
- 1 teaspoon nutmeg, ground
- 1 teaspoon cinnamon powder
- Juice of 1 lime
- 4 tablespoons coconut sugar

Directions:
1. Arrange the bananas in a baking pan, add the nutmeg and the other ingredients, bake at 350 degrees F for 15 minutes.
2. Divide the baked bananas between plates and serve.

Nutrition: calories 206, fat 0.6, fiber 3.2, carbs 47.1, protein 2.4

Cocoa Smoothie

Preparation time: 5 minutes
Cooking time: 0 minutes
Servings: 2

Ingredients:

- 2 teaspoons cocoa powder
- 1 avocado, pitted, peeled and mashed
- 1 cup almond milk
- 1 cup coconut cream

Directions:

1. In your blender, combine the almond milk with the cream and the other ingredients, pulse well, divide in to cups and serve cold.

Nutrition: calories 155, fat 12.3, fiber 4, carbs 8.6, protein 5

Banana Bars

Preparation time: 30 minutes
Cooking time: 0 minutes
Servings: 4
Ingredients:

- 1 cup coconut oil, melted
- 2 bananas, peeled and chopped
- 1 avocado, peeled, pitted and mashed
- ½ cup coconut sugar
- ¼ cup lime juice
- 1 teaspoon lemon zest, grated
- Cooking spray

Directions:

1. In your food processor, mix the bananas with the oil and the other ingredients except the cooking spray and pulse well.
2. Grease a pan with the cooking spray, pour and spread the banana mix, spread, keep in the fridge for 30 minutes, cut into bars and serve.

Nutrition: calories 639, fat 64.6, fiber 4.9, carbs 20.5, protein 1.7

Green Tea and Dates Bars

Preparation time: 10 minutes
Cooking time: 30 minutes
Servings: 8

Ingredients:
- 2 tablespoons green tea powder
- 2 cups coconut milk, heated
- ½ cup coconut oil, melted
- 2 cups coconut sugar
- 4 eggs, whisked
- 2 teaspoons vanilla extract
- 3 cups almond flour
- 1 teaspoon baking soda
- 2 teaspoons baking powder

Directions:
1. In a bowl, combine the coconut milk with the green tea powder and the rest of the ingredients, stir well, pour into a square pan, spread, introduce in the oven, bake at 350 degrees F for 30 minutes, cool down, cut into bars and serve.

Nutrition: calories 560, fat 22.3, fiber 4, carbs 12.8, protein 22.1

Walnut Cream

Preparation time: 2 hours
Cooking time: 0 minutes
Servings: 4

Ingredients:
- 2 cups almond milk
- ½ cup coconut cream
- ½ cup walnuts, chopped
- 3 tablespoons coconut sugar
- 1 teaspoon vanilla extract

Directions:
1. In a bowl, combine the almond milk with the cream and the other ingredients, whisk well, divide into cups and keep in the fridge for 2 hours before serving.

Nutrition: calories 170, fat 12.4, fiber 3, carbs 12.8, protein 4

Lemon Cake

Preparation time: 10 minutes
Cooking time: 35 minutes
Servings: 6

Ingredients:
- 2 cups whole wheat flour
- 1 teaspoon baking powder
- 2 tablespoons coconut oil, melted
- 1 egg, whisked
- 3 tablespoons coconut sugar
- 1 cup almond milk
- Zest of 1 lemon, grated
- Juice of 1 lemon

Directions:
1. In a bowl, combine the flour with the oil and the other ingredients, whisk well, transfer this to a cake pan and bake at 360 degrees F for 35 minutes.
2. Slice and serve cold.

Nutrition: calories 222, fat 12.5, fiber 6.2, carbs 7, protein 17.4

Raisins Bars

Preparation time: 10 minutes
Cooking time: 25 minutes
Servings: 6

Ingredients:
- 1 teaspoon cinnamon powder
- 2 cups almond flour
- 1 teaspoon baking powder
- ½ teaspoon nutmeg, ground
- 1 cup coconut oil, melted
- 1 cup coconut sugar
- 1 egg, whisked
- 1 cup raisins

Directions:
1. In a bowl, combine the flour with the cinnamon and the other ingredients, stir well, spread on a lined baking sheet, introduce in the oven, bake at 380 degrees F for 25 minutes, cut into bars and serve cold.

Nutrition: calories 274, fat 12, fiber 5.2, carbs 14.5, protein 7

Nectarines Squares

Preparation time: 10 minutes
Cooking time: 20 minutes
Servings: 4

Ingredients:
- 3 nectarines, pitted and chopped
- 1 tablespoon coconut sugar
- ½ teaspoon baking soda
- 1 cup almond flour
- 4 tablespoons coconut oil, melted
- 2 tablespoons cocoa powder

Directions:
1. In a blender, combine the nectarines with the sugar and the rest of the ingredients, pulse well, pour into a lined square pan, spread, bake in the oven at 375 degrees F for 20 minutes, leave the mix aside to cool down a bit, cut into squares and serve.

Nutrition: calories 342, fat 14.4, fiber 7.6, carbs 12, protein 7.7

Grapes Stew

Preparation time: 10 minutes
Cooking time: 20 minutes
Servings: 4

Ingredients:
- 1 cup green grapes
- Juice of ½ lime
- 2 tablespoons coconut sugar
- 1 and ½ cups water
- 2 teaspoons cardamom powder

Directions:
1. Heat up a pan with the water medium heat, add the grapes and the other ingredients, bring to a simmer, cook for 20 minutes, divide into bowls and serve.

Nutrition: calories 384, fat 12.5, fiber 6.3, carbs 13.8, protein 5.6

Mandarin and Plums Cream

Preparation time: 10 minutes
Cooking time: 20 minutes
Servings: 4

Ingredients:
- 1 mandarin, peeled and chopped
- ½ pound plums, pitted and chopped
- 1 cup coconut cream
- Juice of 2 mandarins
- 2 tablespoons coconut sugar

Directions:
1. In a blender, combine the mandarin with the plums and the other ingredients, pulse well, divide into small ramekins, introduce in the oven, bake at 350 degrees F for 20 minutes, and serve cold.

Nutrition: calories 402, fat 18.2, fiber 2, carbs 22.2, protein 4.5

Cherry and Strawberries Cream

Preparation time: 10 minutes
Cooking time: 0 minutes
Servings: 6

Ingredients:
- 1 pound cherries, pitted
- 1 cup strawberries, chopped
- ¼ cup coconut sugar
- 2 cups coconut cream

Directions:
1. In a blender, combine the cherries with the other ingredients, pulse well, divide into bowls and serve cold.

Nutrition: calories 342, fat 22.1, fiber 5.6, carbs 8.4, protein 6.5

Cardamom Walnuts and Rice Pudding

Preparation time: 5 minutes
Cooking time: 40 minutes
Servings: 4

Ingredients:
- 1 cup basmati rice
- 3 cups almond milk
- 3 tablespoons coconut sugar
- ½ teaspoon cardamom powder
- ¼ cup walnuts, chopped

Directions:
1. In a pan, combine the rice with the milk and the other ingredients, stir, cook for 40 minutes over medium heat, divide into bowls and serve cold.

Nutrition: calories 703, fat 47.9, fiber 5.2, carbs 62.1, protein 10.1

Pears Bread

Preparation time: 10 minutes
Cooking time: 30 minutes
Servings: 4

Ingredients:
- 2 cups pears, cored and cubed
- 1 cup coconut sugar
- 2 eggs, whisked
- 2 cups almond flour
- 1 tablespoon baking powder
- 1 tablespoon coconut oil, melted

Directions:
1. In a bowl, mix the pears with the sugar and the other ingredients, whisk, pour into a loaf pan, introduce in the oven and bake at 350 degrees F for 30 minutes.
2. Slice and serve cold.

Nutrition: calories 380, fat 16.7, fiber 5, carbs 17.5, protein 5.6

Rice and Cherries Pudding

Preparation time: 10 minutes
Cooking time: 25 minutes
Servings: 4

Ingredients:
- 1 tablespoon coconut oil, melted
- 1 cup white rice
- 3 cups almond milk
- ½ cup cherries, pitted and halved
- 3 tablespoons coconut sugar
- 1 teaspoon cinnamon powder
- 1 teaspoon vanilla extract

Directions:
1. In a pan, combine the oil with the rice and the other ingredients, stir, bring to a simmer, cook for 25 minutes over medium heat, divide into bowls and serve cold.

Nutrition: calories 292, fat 12.4, fiber 5.6, carbs 8, protein 7

Watermelon Stew

Preparation time: 5 minutes
Cooking time: 8 minutes
Servings: 4

Ingredients:
- Juice of 1 lime
- 1 teaspoon lime zest, grated
- 1 and ½ cup coconut sugar
- 4 cups watermelon, peeled and cut into large chunks
- 1 and ½ cups water

Directions:
1. In a pan, combine the watermelon with the lime zest, and the other ingredients, toss, bring to a simmer over medium heat, cook for 8 minutes, divide into bowls and serve cold.

Nutrition:: calories 233, fat 0.2, fiber 0.7, carbs 61.5, protein 0.9

Ginger Pudding

Preparation time: 1 hour
Cooking time: 0 minutes
Servings: 4

Ingredients:
- 2 cups almond milk
- ½ cup coconut cream
- 2 tablespoons coconut sugar
- 1 tablespoon ginger, grated
- ¼ cup chia seeds

Directions:
1. In a bowl, combine the milk with the cream and the other ingredients, whisk well, divide into small cups and keep them in the fridge for 1 hour before serving.

Nutrition: calories 345, fat 17, fiber 4.7, carbs 11.5, protein 6.9

Cashew Cream

Preparation time: 2 hours
Cooking time: 0 minutes
Servings: 4

Ingredients:
- 1 cup cashews, chopped
- 2 tablespoons coconut oil, melted
- 2 tablespoons coconut oil, melted
- 1 cup coconut cream
- tablespoons lemon juice
- 1 tablespoons coconut sugar

Directions:
1. In a blender, combine the cashews with the coconut oil and the other ingredients, pulse well, divide into small cups and keep in the fridge for 2 hours before serving.

Nutrition: calories 480, fat 43.9, fiber 2.4, carbs 19.7, protein 7

Hemp Cookies

Preparation time: 30 minutes
Cooking time: 0 minutes
Servings: 6

Ingredients:
- 1 cup almonds, soaked overnight and drained
- 2 tablespoons cocoa powder
- 1 tablespoon coconut sugar
- ½ cup hemp seeds
- ¼ cup coconut, shredded
- ½ cup water

Directions:
1. In your food processor, combine the almonds with the cocoa powder and the other ingredients, pulse well, press this on a lined baking sheet, keep in the fridge for 30 minutes, slice and serve.

Nutrition: calories 270, fat 12.6, fiber 3, carbs 7.7, protein 7

Almonds and Pomegranate Bowls

Preparation time: 2 hours
Cooking time: 0 minutes
Servings: 4

Ingredients:
- ½ cup coconut cream
- 1 teaspoon vanilla extract
- 1 cup almonds, chopped
- 1 cup pomegranate seeds
- 1 tablespoon coconut sugar

Directions:
1. In a bowl, combine the almonds with the cream and the other ingredients, toss, divide into small bowls and serve.

Nutrition: calories 258, fat 19, fiber 3.9, carbs 17.6, protein 6.2

www.ingramcontent.com/pod-product-compliance
Lightning Source LLC
Chambersburg PA
CBHW071817080526
44589CB00012B/822